Ligaments of the Knee

Alfred J. Tria Jr. • Giles R. Scuderi
Editors

Ligaments of the Knee

A Machine-Generated Literature Overview

Springer

Editors
Alfred J. Tria Jr.
Department of Orthopedics
Rutgers-Robert Wood Johnson
Medical School
New Brunswick, NJ, USA

Giles R. Scuderi
Northwell Health Orthopaedic Institute
New York, NY, USA

ISBN 978-3-031-66617-9 ISBN 978-3-031-66615-5 (eBook)
https://doi.org/10.1007/978-3-031-66615-5

This Springer imprint is published by the registered company Springer Nature Switzerland AG
The registered company address is: Gewerbestrasse 11, 6330 Cham, Switzerland

Ligaments of the Knee

Auto-summaries can be generated by either an abstractive or extractive auto-summarization:

- An extraction-based summarizer identifies the most important sentences of a text and uses the original sentences to create the summary.
- An abstraction-based summarizer creates new text based on deep learning. New phrases are created to summarize the content.

The auto-summaries you will find in this book have been generated via an abstractive summarization approach.

Each chapter was carefully edited by Dr. Alfred J. Tria Jr., and Dr. Giles R. Scuderi. The editors selected the papers which were then auto-summarized. The editors have not edited the auto-summaries due to the extraction-based approach and have not changed the original sentences. You will find the editors' reviews and guidance on the auto-summaries in their chapter introductions.

In machine-generated books, editors are defined as those who curate the content for the book by selecting the papers to be auto-summarized and by organizing the output into a meaningful order. Next to the thoughtful curation of the papers, editors should guide the readers through the auto-summaries and make transparent why they selected the papers.

The ultimate goal is to provide a current literature review of Springer Nature publications on a given topic in order to support readers in overcoming information overload and to help them dive into a topic faster; to identify interdisciplinary overlaps; and to present papers which might not have been on the readers' radar.

Please note that the selected papers are not used to train an LLM while the auto-summaries are created.

Preface

> Dig deep; the water-goodness-is down there. And as long as you keep digging, it will keep bubbling up.
> Marcus Aurelius (Meditations, Book 7, article 59)

Every orthopedic surgeon, anatomist, and biomechanical engineer has had to consider the ligaments of the knee at some point in his or her career. This begins in medical school for the orthopedist and continues through residency training and clinical practice. For some it may have been a passing item on the way to another subspecialty and for others it forms a center of interest and challenge. Ligament injuries are common in today's societies with the emphasis on exercise and sports contests.

The literature has expanded in an exponential fashion making it more difficult to review the pertinent items and to summarize them in an appropriate manner.

Artificial Intelligence (AI) has become more and more a part of our everyday experience with some enthusiastic acceptance and some doubts and fears. As with the computers we use every day, AI can help with some of the most tedious endeavors but is still dependent upon human intervention and suggestion.

The purpose of this book is to generate the pertinent articles for each of the ligament sections by submitting keywords and then, asking the machines to generate keywords and articles. This is then reviewed by the editors and returned for machine-generated summaries. This machine-generated literature overview only considers articles published by Springer Nature. Perhaps, in the future it may be possible to widen the overview with appropriate guidelines when the challenges of intellectual property can be overcome.

The editors hope that this will be an early example of the assistance that AI can afford investigators in searching the literature and advancing academic information.

New Brunswick, NJ, USA — Alfred J. Tria Jr.
New York, NY, USA — Giles R. Scuderi

Contents

Part IV Surgery

About the Editor

Alfred J. Tria Jr. MD is the Emeritus Clinical Professor of Orthopedic Surgery from the Department of Orthopedic Surgery at Rutgers-Robert Wood Johnson Medical School in New Brunswick, New Jersey. He received his AB from Harvard College and his MD from Harvard Medical School. He did his residency training at Columbia University in New York City and completed his Knee Fellowship at The Hospital for Special Surgery with Dr. John N. Insall. He is a member of The Knee Society and the American Association of Hip and Knee Surgeons. He has published more than 200 articles and 20 textbooks. His special interest is in knee arthroplasty and he patented "Minimally invasive Total Knee Arthroplasty Method and Instrumentation."

Giles R. Scuderi MD is Vice President of the Orthopedic Service Line at Northwell Health in New York, Professor of Orthopedic Surgery at Zucker School of Medicine at Hofstra/Northwell, Fellowship Director of Adult Reconstruction at Lenox Hill Hospital in New York City, and attending orthopedic surgeon at Lenox Hill Hospital and Long Island Jewish Valley Stream Hospital. His practice focuses on adult knee reconstruction, total knee arthroplasty, and revision knee surgery. He has published extensively in numerous orthopedic journals, edited numerous text books, and continues to lecture worldwide. Dr. Scuderi is a past president of The Knee Society, a member of the American Association of Hip and Knee Surgeons and the Arthroscopy Association of North America.

Part I
Anatomy

1.1 Introduction by the Editor

The references in this chapter are searched by using key words that are chosen by the [GR1] editors. The words are submitted to computers that in turn list a set of AI generated key words and refences from the Springer Network. The editors, then, review the selected articles to determine if they are appropriate for the section and return them for AI summaries. The summaries from AI are, then, reviewed by the editors for wording and grammar. The search for bibliographies is much broader because it is not limited to the Springer Network. However, not all of those chosen articles can be summarized. After the final review by the editors, the manuscript is returned for production.

The knee joint consists of three articulations: medial tibio-femoral, lateral tibio-femoral, and patellofemoral. The range of motion (ROM) is controlled by the articular surfaces and the surrounding ligaments.

There are four major ligaments: anterior cruciate ligament (ACL), posterior cruciate ligament (PCL), medial collateral ligament (MCL), and lateral collateral ligament (LCL). There are multiple accessory ligaments. Anteriorly, the medial and lateral patellofemoral ligaments assist in patellar tracking. Posteriorly, there are the ligaments of Humphrey and Wrisberg that are anterior and posterior to the PCL respectively. The posterior oblique ligament and the oblique popliteal ligament are posteromedial and the arcuate ligament and the fabellofibular ligament are posterolateral.

The cruciate ligaments are the major contributors to anterior/posterior stability. The femoral origins and the tibial insertions have been thoroughly studied and are critical for surgical reconstructions of the torn ligaments. They are each two bundle structures, while some investigators suggest that the ACL has three bundles. The spiral nature of the ligaments contributes to the complex rotation of the knee joint throughout the ROM.

The ACL is the least robust of the two cruciates and is more commonly injured, especially in sports activities. There are six articles reviewed in this section).

Duthon's article illustrates that the cross-sectional area changes along its length and the variable strain adaptation make replication of the anatomy difficult. Bicer confirmed that there are two bundles and studied the origins and insertions which should help with anatomic reconstruction. Fugie's article proposes three bundles but this may be over dissection of the ligament. There are a multitude of approaches that address tears of the ACL: primary repairs, autograft reconstructions, allograft reconstructions, and synthetic augmentations. All of these techniques are affected by the anatomic articles in this section. The classic references in the bibliography are written by Kennedy (nerve supply), Girgis (anatomical function), Arnoczky (anatomy), and Scapinelli (vascular anatomy).

The PCL is less commonly injured; and, in the past, tears of the ligament often went undiagnosed. With more modern evaluation techniques and clinical awareness, the literature has more articles addressing anatomy and surgical approaches. Six articles are summarized in this section. Logterman reviews the function of the two bundles. Fugie proposes an anatomic landmark (the dimple) for ligament reconstruction. Verhey proposes an anatomic variant, but once again, this may represent over dissection. The classic references in the bibliography are written by Girgis (anatomy), Woo (tensile properties), and Scapinelli (vascular anatomy.)

The collateral ligaments (MCL and LCL) are the major supports to valgus and varus stress. They are typically injured when the knee is subjected to a stress in the coronal plane of the joint along with some rotational component that injures the collateral ligaments along with an associated cruciate ligament.

The MCL section has seven references. Sanghvi, Kuriyama, and Tsutsumi delve into the anatomy of the posterior oblique ligament and its importance in knee injuries. The classic references in the bibliography are written by Hughston (role of the posterior oblique ligament), Brantigan (anatomy), and Warren (supporting structures medially).

Chapter 1
The Anterior Cruciate Ligament

Alfred J. Tria Jr. and Giles R. Scuderi

Introduction by the Editor

The anterior cruciate ligament (ACL) is a central stabilizer of the knee that prevents anterior motion in both full extension and 90 degrees of flexion. It is embryologically present by 6 weeks of gestation [5]. Its blood supply is from the middle geniculate. Scapinelli confirmed this with his autopsy dissections and contrast injections. There is minimal supply from the bone origin or insertion [33]. Schutte et al. identified mechanoreceptors and free nerve endings that account for motion, speed, acceleration, and pain reception. The innervations account for proprioception [36]. The double bundle structure enables the ligament to stabilize the knee throughout the range of motion [92].

Machine Generated Summaries

Disclaimer: The summaries in this chapter were generated from Springer Nature publications using abstractive AI auto-summarization: An abstraction-based summarizer creates new text based on deep learning. New phrases are created to summarize the content. As the constituted sentences are machine selected, they may not fully reflect the body of the work, so we strongly advise that the original content is read and cited. The auto-generated summaries were curated by the editor to meet Springer Nature publication standards.

A. J. Tria Jr. (✉)
Department of Orthopedics, Rutgers-Robert Wood Johnson Medical School, New Brunswick, NJ, USA

G. R. Scuderi
Northwell Health Orthopaedic Institute, New York, NY, USA

A. J. Tria Jr., G. R. Scuderi (eds.), *Ligaments of the Knee*,
https://doi.org/10.1007/978-3-031-66615-5_1

Machine generated keywords: footprint, mri, femoral, bundle, age, tibial, attachment, femoral attachment, tibial footprint, anatomic, acl, femoral footprint, force, acl femoral, double bundle.

Anatomy of the Anterior Cruciate Ligament [92]

This is a machine-generated summary of:

Duthon, V. B.; Barea, C.; Abrassart, S.; Fasel, J. H.; Fritschy, D.; Ménétrey, J.: Anatomy of the anterior cruciate ligament [92]

Published in: Knee Surgery, Sports Traumatology, Arthroscopy (2005)

Link to original: https://doi.org/10.1007/s00167-005-0679-9

If you want to cite the papers, please refer to the original.

For technical reasons we could not place the page where the original quote is coming from.

Research Highlights

The anterior cruciate ligament (ACL) is a critical component of the knee joint, essential for maintaining stability during dynamic movements. Despite its importance, the ACL's intricate anatomy and biomechanics are not fully understood, particularly in relation to its healing potential and surgical reconstruction. A study by Duthon et al. presents a systematic review of the macroanatomy, microanatomy, and biomechanical function of the ACL, providing insights that could enhance clinical outcomes for ACL injuries.

Duthon et al. compiled data from various original research studies to construct a comprehensive picture of the ACL's structure and function. They examined the ligament's development from embryonic stages through to its complex adult form, which includes variations in cross-sectional shape and area along its length. The study delved into the functional differentiation within the ACL, such as the division into anteromedial and posterolateral bundles, which exhibit distinct patterns of length changes during knee movement. The researchers also explored the microanatomy of the ACL, revealing zones with varying cellular compositions and collagen types that reflect the ligament's exposure to different mechanical stresses. By integrating findings on innervation and vascularization, Duthon et al. shed light on factors influencing the ACL's limited healing capacity.

The main advances highlighted by Duthon et al.'s research include a detailed understanding of the ACL's complex structural organization and its implications for surgical reconstruction. The study emphasizes that replicating the original anatomy and biomechanics of the ACL remains challenging due to its unique properties, such as multi-axial stress resistance and variable tensile strain adaptation. Looking forward, these insights could guide improvements in ACL repair techniques, aiming to better mimic natural ligament function and potentially preserve proprioception post-reconstruction. As Duthon et al. suggest, future research may focus on optimizing surgical methods to accommodate the intricate anatomy and biomechanics of the ACL, enhancing patient outcomes after injury.

Current Knowledge in the Anatomy of the Human Anterior Cruciate Ligament [93]

This is a machine-generated summary of:

Bicer, Elcil Kaya; Lustig, Sebastien; Servien, Elvire; Selmi, Tarık Ait Si; Neyret, Philippe: Current knowledge in the anatomy of the human anterior cruciate ligament [93]

Published in: Knee Surgery, Sports Traumatology, Arthroscopy (2009)

Link to original: https://doi.org/10.1007/s00167-009-0993-8

If you want to cite the papers, please refer to the original.

For technical reasons we could not place the page where the original quote is coming from.

Research Highlights

The anterior cruciate ligament (ACL) is a critical component in maintaining knee stability, yet its complex anatomy and function continue to challenge orthopedic surgeons. Despite extensive research, there remains a lack of consensus on the optimal surgical techniques for ACL reconstruction. A study by Bicer et al. delves into the macro and ultrastructural properties of the ACL, providing insights into its insertion sites and associated landmarks that could enhance surgical precision and outcomes.

Bicer et al. meticulously dissected fetal and adult knee specimens to elucidate the detailed anatomy of the ACL. They employed a variety of methods including histological examination, which revealed differences in cellular composition between fetal and adult ACLs, as well as anatomic dissections that confirmed the presence of two distinct bundles within the ligament. The study also investigated the femoral and tibial insertion sites, uncovering variations in shape and size that have significant implications for surgical reconstruction. By integrating embryological development with gross anatomical observations, the authors offer a nuanced understanding of ACL structure that underscores the importance of individualized surgical approaches.

Mechanical Functions of the Three Bundles Consisting of the Human Anterior Cruciate Ligament [94]

This is a machine-generated summary of:

Fujie, H.; Otsubo, H.; Fukano, S.; Suzuki, T.; Suzuki, D.; Mae, T.; Shino, K.: Mechanical functions of the three bundles consisting of the human anterior cruciate ligament [94]

Published in: Knee Surgery, Sports Traumatology, Arthroscopy (2011)

Link to original: https://doi.org/10.1007/s00167-011-1513-1

If you want to cite the papers, please refer to the original.

For technical reasons we could not place the page where the original quote is coming from.

Research Highlights

The evolution of anterior cruciate ligament (ACL) reconstruction techniques, particularly the shift from single-bundle to double- and triple-bundle reconstructions, has been driven by a desire to more closely mimic the ACL's natural anatomy and biomechanics. Despite advancements, there remains a knowledge gap in understanding the precise biomechanical functions of the ACL's individual bundles during various knee movements. Now a new study by Fujie et al. addresses this gap by investigating the force distribution among the anteromedial medial (AMM), anteromedial lateral (AML), and posterolateral (PL) bundles of the human ACL in response to different knee motions using a 6-DOF robotic system.

Fujie et al. employed a six-axis manipulator integrated with a six-degree-of-freedom universal force/moment sensor to analyze cadaveric knees. This allowed to simulate natural knee motion while precisely measuring the forces on each ACL bundle. The team prepared five human cadaveric knees, ensuring intact ligaments and absence of degenerative disease, to establish accurate baseline measurements. They then subjected these knees to hyperextension, passive flexion-extension, and anterior force application while recording detailed kinematic and kinetic data.

The methodology involved dividing the ACL into its constituent bundles and measuring their cross-sectional areas. The researchers then sequentially transected each bundle to isolate their individual contributions to knee stability. By reproducing intact knee motion on our robotic system after each transection, they could determine the force each bundle resists during different movements. This innovative approach allowed for an unprecedented look at how each part of the ACL responds to stress, revealing that the AMM bundle plays a pivotal role across a wide range of motion.

The study demonstrates that the AMM bundle is the primary stabilizer against anterior tibial translation throughout most knee movements, while the AML bundle becomes more important at deeper flexion angles. Conversely, the PL bundle is essential for resisting hyperextension and stabilizing the knee at full extension. Their insights are crucial for refining ACL reconstruction techniques, as they underscore the importance of restoring each bundle's function to achieve optimal joint stability. Looking forward, this research sets a foundation for future studies that could explore rotational stability and other complex loading scenarios, further enhancing ACL reconstruction strategies and patient outcomes.

Anterior Cruciate Ligament Femoral Footprint Is Oblong-Ovate, Triangular, or Two-Tears Shaped in Healthy Young Adults: Three-Dimensional MRI Analysis [95]

This is a machine-generated summary of:

Lin, Jinrong; Zhang, Shurong; Xin, Enhui; Liang, Meng; Yang, Liqin; Chen, Jiwu: Anterior cruciate ligament femoral footprint is oblong-ovate, triangular, or two-tears shaped in healthy young adults: three-dimensional MRI analysis [95]

Published in: Knee Surgery, Sports Traumatology, Arthroscopy (2023)

Link to original: https://doi.org/10.1007/s00167-023-07606-6

If you want to cite the papers, please refer to the original.

For technical reasons we could not place the page where the original quote is coming from.

Research Highlights

Anterior cruciate ligament (ACL) injuries are a common affliction, particularly among athletes, leading to surgical intervention through ACL reconstruction (ACLR). Despite advancements in surgical techniques, failure rates remain high, often due to errors such as inaccurate femoral tunnel placement. A detailed understanding of the ACL femoral footprint is helpful for improving ACLR outcomes. A study by Lin et al. has leveraged high-resolution magnetic resonance imaging (MRI) to assess the morphology of the ACL femoral footprint with precision, revealing three distinct shapes with significant variations in location.

Lin et al. conducted their research on subjects with healthy knees, using a 3.0 T MR system and advanced imaging sequences to evaluate the ACL. The post-processing involved identifying the ligament's insertion site and measuring various anatomical features associated with ACL injury risk. The researchers employed

Materialise's Interactive Medical Image Control System software for reconstructive modeling, ensuring measurement precision within millimeters. Their approach achieved substantial intra- and inter-observer reliability in defining the footprint's shape, size, and location.

The study's main advance is the categorization of the ACL femoral footprint into three distinct shapes: oblong-ovate (OO), two-tears (TT), and a third shape resembling a semicircle (Tr). Despite similar areas across these types, their locations varied significantly, suggesting that a universal approach to ACLR may not be optimal. The TT-shaped footprint was associated with characteristics that might predispose individuals to ACL injuries, warranting further investigation into clinical implications. Moreover, this research challenges previous findings by demonstrating similar areas between different footprint shapes and suggesting that double-bundle ACLR could offer better coverage of the native footprint compared to single-bundle techniques.

In conclusion, Lin et al. provides insights into the morphology of the ACL femoral footprint using MRI technology. By accurately identifying three distinct shapes and their respective locations, this research underscores the need for personalized surgical planning in ACLR. While acknowledging limitations such as sample size and demographic scope, future research directions include expanding participant diversity and exploring variations in patients with ACL tears.

The Morphology of the Tibial Footprint of the Anterior Cruciate Ligament Changes with Ageing from Oval/Elliptical to C-Shaped [96]

This is a machine-generated summary of:

Morales-Avalos, Rodolfo; Castillo-Escobedo, Tadeo A.; Elizondo-Omaña, Rodrigo E.; del Carmen Theriot-Giron, María; Perelli, Simone; Guzmán-López, Santos; Peña-Martínez, Víctor M.; Vílchez-Cavazos, Félix; Monllau, Juan Carlos: The morphology of the tibial footprint of the anterior cruciate ligament changes with ageing from oval/elliptical to C-shaped [96]

Published in: Knee Surgery, Sports Traumatology, Arthroscopy (2020)

Link to original: https://doi.org/10.1007/s00167-020-06049-7

If you want to cite the papers, please refer to the original.

For technical reasons we could not place the page where the original quote is coming from.

Research Highlights

Anterior cruciate ligament (ACL) injuries are common, particularly among young, active individuals, and ACL reconstruction aims to closely replicate the native ligament's anatomy to restore knee function and prevent long-term issues like osteoarthritis. Despite the known importance of accurately reconstructing the ACL's tibial footprint, its shape remains a subject of debate, with various morphologies described and no standardized classification system. A study by Morales-Avalos et al. addresses this knowledge gap by examining the morphological changes in the ACL tibial footprint with aging in healthy knees, hypothesizing that age-related degenerative processes alter its shape.

The research conducted by Morales-Avalos et al. was an anatomical, observational study reviewing 400 nonpaired, formalin-fixed human cadaver knees of Mexican descent. The specimens were divided into age and gender groups for analysis. Exclusion criteria ensured that only knees without significant pathology were studied.

Dissections were performed to expose the ACL's tibial footprints. High-resolution digital photographs documented each specimen for further evaluation. Three independent observers, blinded to specimen details, assessed the morphology using a previously proposed classification system. Statistical analyses included intra- and inter-observer reliability checks and comparisons across age and gender groups.

The study's main advance is the confirmation that the ACL's tibial footprint morphology does indeed vary with age, transitioning from an oval/elliptical shape in younger specimens to a "C" shape in older specimens. This finding suggests a physiological degeneration process predominantly affecting the posterolateral bundle of the ACL over time.

These observations have significant clinical implications for ACL reconstruction techniques, which may need to be tailored based on patient age to ensure accurate restoration of the ligament's footprint. The research sets a foundation for future studies to explore how these morphological changes impact knee biomechanics and surgical outcomes across different populations. As Morales-Avalos et al. suggest, understanding these variations can lead to more individualized surgical approaches that minimize damage to surrounding structures and improve long-term joint health.

Evaluation of Age-Related Differences in Anterior Cruciate Ligament Size [97]

This is a machine-generated summary of:

Iriuchishima, Takanori; Ryu, Keinosuke; Fu, Freddie H.: Evaluation of age-related differences in anterior cruciate ligament size [97]

Published in: Knee Surgery, Sports Traumatology, Arthroscopy (2018)

Link to original: https://doi.org/10.1007/s00167-018-5336-1

Copyright of the summarized publication:

If you want to cite the papers, please refer to the original.

For technical reasons we could not place the page where the original quote is coming from.

Research Highlights

The anterior cruciate ligament (ACL) is critical for knee stability, particularly in young, active individuals. Anatomical ACL reconstruction aims to restore knee function by replicating the ligament's natural anatomy. Despite advancements, there is still debate over the precise anatomical details of the ACL and the optimal placement of tunnels during reconstruction. This uncertainty is compounded by the use of elderly cadaveric knees in studies, which may not accurately represent the ACL morphology in younger populations who are more likely to require reconstruction. Iriuchishima et al. addresses this knowledge gap by examining the relationship between age and in vivo ACL morphological characteristics using magnetic resonance imaging (MRI), challenging the assumption that ACL size diminishes with age.

Iriuchishima et al. conducted a retrospective analysis using MRI data to compare ACL size in young and elderly subjects. The young group consisted of individuals under a certain age with meniscus injuries but intact ACLs, while the elderly group comprised subjects over a certain age undergoing evaluation before unicompartmental knee arthroplasty without significant osteoarthritis or ACL deterioration. The researchers measured axial and sagittal ACL sizes, as well as various aspects of knee bony morphology, using a PACS system with high measurement accuracy. They normalized ACL areas against knee bony morphology to account for differences in knee size.

The study revealed that while sagittal ACL size was significantly larger in younger subjects, no difference was found when normalized for knee bony morphology between young and elderly groups. This suggests that differences in body and knee size, rather than age-related atrophy, may account for variations in ACL size. The authors highlight that these findings have implications for both surgical practice and anatomical research.

The study by Iriuchishima et al. provides insights into the impact of aging on ACL morphology. It demonstrates a significant negative correlation between age and sagittal ACL size but shows that this does not necessarily indicate an age-related decline when considering proportional differences in knee and body size. These findings underscore the importance of considering individual anatomical variations during ACL reconstruction, particularly in elderly patients. Iriuchishima reported that when performing ACL reconstruction on older patients or using cadaveric knees from older individuals for anatomical studies, it is crucial to take into account these size differences. Future research should expand on these findings with larger sample sizes and diverse ethnic groups to further refine our understanding of ACL anatomy across different populations.

2D and 3D 3-Tesla Magnetic Resonance Imaging of the Double Bundle Structure in Anterior Cruciate Ligament Anatomy [98]

This is a machine-generated summary of:

Steckel, Hanno; Vadala, Gianluca; Davis, Denise; Fu, Freddie H.: 2D and 3D 3-tesla magnetic resonance imaging of the double bundle structure in anterior cruciate ligament anatomy [98]

Published in: Knee Surgery, Sports Traumatology, Arthroscopy (2006)

Link to original: https://doi.org/10.1007/s00167-006-0185-8

If you want to cite the papers, please refer to the original.

For technical reasons we could not place the page where the original quote is coming from.

Research Highlights

Magnetic Resonance Imaging (MRI) has become the gold standard for diagnosing anterior cruciate ligament (ACL) injuries, offering detailed insights into normal and pathological ACL anatomy. Despite advancements in MRI technology, challenges persist in evaluating partial ACL tears and the double bundle structure, which is crucial for preoperative planning in ACL reconstruction surgery. A study by Steckel et al. aims to assess the ability of 7-T ultra-high-field strength MRI to distinguish the double bundle structure of the ACL in human cadaver knees.

The observational non-clinical study by Steckel et al. utilized six cadaver knees to explore the ACL anatomy using a 7-T MRI scanner. The researchers selected imaging protocols, including various pulsing sequences and multiplanar imaging, to optimize visualization of the anteromedial (AM) and posterolateral (PL) bundles of the ACL. By employing a combination of sagittal, oblique coronal, and oblique sagittal proton-density-weighted fast spin echo sequences, they achieved high-resolution images that highlighted the distinct anatomy of each bundle. The team's innovative use of a custom-built extremity coil demonstrated superior sensitivity and signal-to-noise ratio compared to standard coils. Following MRI scans, arthroscopic validation confirmed the accuracy of their imaging findings, establishing a strong correlation between MRI observations and macroscopic anatomy.

This study represents an advance in MRI diagnostics for ACL injuries, demonstrating that 7-T ultra-high-field strength MRI can effectively differentiate between the AM and PL bundles of the ACL. This information can potentially allow surgeons to tailor reconstructions based on the individual status of each bundle. Future research should focus on applying these findings in a clinical setting to improve patient outcomes. By refining imaging protocols further and correlating them with clinical data, this research paves the way for more precise preoperative assessments and could lead to more targeted and efficient rehabilitation protocols.

Bibliography

1. Beynnon BD, Johnson RJ, Fleming BC, et al. The effect of functional knee bracing on the anterior cruciate ligament in the weightbearing and non-weightbearing knee. Am J Sports Med. 1997;25:353–9.
2. Matsumoto H, Suda Y, Otani T, et al. Roles of the anterior cruciate ligament and the medial collateral ligament in preventing valgus instability. J Orthop Sci. 2001;6:28–32.
3. Sakane M, Fox RJ, Woo SL-Y, Livesay GA, Li G, Fu F. In situ forces in the anterior cruciate ligament and its bundles in response to anterior tibial loads. J Orthop Res. 1997;15:285–93.
4. Bach BR Jr, Levy ME, Bojchuk J, Tradonsky S, Bush-Joseph CA, Khan NH. Single-incision endoscopic anterior cruciate ligament reconstruction using patellar tendon autograft. Minimum two-year follow-up evaluation. Am J Sports Med. 1998;26:30–40.
5. Ellison AE, Berg EE. Embryology, anatomy, and function of the anterior cruciate ligament. Orthop Clin North Am. 1985;16:3–14.
6. Bernard M, Hertel P, Hornung H, et al. Femoral insertion of the anterior cruciate ligament. Radiographic quadrant method. Am J Knee Surg. 1997;10:14–22.
7. Amis AA, Dawkins GPC. Functional anatomy of the anterior cruciate ligament. Fibre bundle actions related to ligament replacements and injuries. J Bone Joint Surg. 1991;73(B):260–7.
8. Amiel D, Billings E, Akeson WH. Ligament structure, chemistry and physiology. In: Daniel D, et al., editors. Knee ligaments: structure, function, injury and repair. New York: Raven Press; 1989. p. 34.
9. Benjamin M, Evans EJ. Fibrocartilage. J Anat. 1990;171:1–15.
10. Koch S, Tillman B. The distal tendon of biceps brachis. Ann Anat. 1995;177:467–74.
11. Kennedy JC, Alexander IJ, Hayes KC. Nerve supply of the human knee and its functional importance. Am J Sports Med. 1982;10:329–35.
12. Konishi Y, Fukubayashi T, Takeshita D. Possible mechanism of quadriceps femoris weakness in patients with ruptured anterior cruciate ligament. Med Sci Sports Exerc. 2002;34:1414–8.
13. Krogsgaard MR, Dyhre-Poulsen P, Fischer-Rasmussen T. Cruciate ligament reflexes. J Electromyogr Kinesiol. 2002;12:177–82.
14. Konishi Y, Suzuki Y, Hirose N, Fukubayashi T. Effects of lidocaine into knee on QF strength and EMG in patients with ACL lesion. Med Sci Sports Exerc. 2003;35:1805–8.
15. Beynnon BD, Fleming BC, Labovitch R, Parsons B. Chronic anterior cruciate ligament deficiency is associated with increased anterior translation of the tibia during the transition from non-weightbearing to weightbearing. J Orthop Res. 2002;20:332–7.
16. Beynnon BD, Pope MH, Wertheimer CM, et al. The effect of functional knee-braces on strain on the anterior cruciate ligament in vivo. J Bone Joint Surg. 1992;74A:1298–312.
17. Beynnon BD, Johnson RJ. Relevant biomechanics. In: DeLee JC, Drez D, editors. Orthopaedic sports medicine; 1994. p. 1113–33.
18. Woo SL-Y, Hollis M, Adams DJ, et al. Tensile properties of the human femur-anterior cruciate ligament–tibia complex. The effects of specimen age and orientation. Am J Sports Med. 1991;19:217–25.
19. Mérida-Velasco JA, Sánchez-Montesinos I, Espín-Ferra J, Mérida-Velasco JR, Rodríguez-Vázquez JF, Jiménez-Collado J. Development of the human knee joint ligaments. Anat Rec. 1997;248:259–68.
20. Ratajczak W. Early development of the cruciate ligaments in staged human embryos in staged human embryos. Folia Morphol. 2000;59:285–90.
21. Tena-Arregui J, Barrio-Asensio C, Viejo-Tirado F, Puerta-Fonollá J, Murillo-González J. Arthroscopic study of the knee joint in fetuses. Arthroscopy. 2003;19:862–8.
22. Harner CD, Baek GH, Vogrin TM, Carlin GJ, Kashiwaguchi S, Woo SL. Quantitative analysis of human cruciate ligament insertions. Arthroscopy. 1999;15:741–9.
23. Siebold R, Ellert T, Metz S, Metz J. Tibial insertions of the anteromedial and posterolateral bundles of the anterior cruciate ligament: morphometry, arthroscopic landmarks, and orientation model for bone tunnel placement. Arthroscopy. 2008;24:154–61.

24. Girgis FG, Marshall JL, Monajem A. The cruciate ligaments of the knee joint. Anatomical, functional and experimental analysis. Clin Orthop Relat Res. 1975;106:216–31.
25. Zantop T, Petersen W, Fu FH. Anatomy of the anterior cruciate ligament. Oper Tech Orthop. 2005;15:20–8.
26. Petersen W, Tillmann B. Anatomy and function of the anterior cruciate ligament. Orthopäde. 2002;31:710–8.
27. Hollis JM, Takai S, Adams DJ, Horibe S, Woo SL. The effects of knee motion and external loading on the length of the anterior cruciate ligament (ACL): a kinematic study. J Biomech Eng. 1991;113:208–14.
28. Takai S, Woo SL, Livesay GA, Adams DJ, Fu FH. Determination of the in situ loads on the human anterior cruciate ligament. J Orthop Res. 1993;11:686–95.
29. Amis AA, Dawkins GPC. Functional anatomy of the anterior cruciate ligament: fibre bundle actions related to ligament replacements and injuries. J Bone Joint Surg Br. 1991;73B:260–7.
30. Petersen W, Tillmann B. Structure and vascularization of the cruciate ligaments of the human knee joint. Anat Embryol (Berl). 1999;200:325–34.
31. Strocchi R, de Pasquale V, Gubellini P, Facchini A, Marcacci M, Buda R, Zaffagnini S, Ruggeri A. The human anterior cruciate ligament: histological and ultrastructural observations. J Anat. 1992;180:515–9.
32. Arnoczky SP. Anatomy of the anterior cruciate ligament. Clin Orthop Relat Res. 1983;172:19–25.
33. Scapinelli R. Vascular anatomy of the human cruciate ligaments and surrounding structures. Clin Anat. 1997;10:151–62.
34. Duthon VB, Barea C, Abrassart S, Fasel JH, Fritschy D, Ménétrey J. Anatomy of the anterior cruciate ligament. Knee Surg Sports Traumatol Arthrosc. 2006;14:204–13.
35. Schultz RA, Miller DC, Kerr CS, Micheli L. Mechanoreceptors in human cruciate ligaments. A histological study. J Bone Joint Surg Am. 1984;66:1072–6.
36. Schutte MJ, Dabezies EJ, Zimny ML, Happel LT. Neural anatomy of the human anterior cruciate ligament. J Bone Joint Surg Am. 1987;69:243–7.
37. Georgoulis AD, Pappa L, Moebius U, Malamou-Mitsi V, Pappa S, Papageorgiou CO, Agnantis NJ, Soucacos PN. The presence of proprioceptive mechanoreceptors in the remnants of the ruptured ACL as a possible source of re-innervation of the ACL autograft. Knee Surg Sports Traumatol Arthrosc. 2001;9:364–8.
38. Adachi N, Ochi M, Uchio Y, Iwasa J, Ryoke K, Kuriwaka M. Mechanoreceptors in the anterior cruciate ligament contribute to the joint position sense. Acta Orthop Scand. 2002;73:330–4.
39. Zarins B, Rowe CR. Combined anterior cruciate ligament reconstruction using semitendinosus tendon and iliotibial tract. J Bone Joint Surg Am. 1986;68:160–77.
40. Friederich NF, O'Brien WR. Anterior cruciate ligament graft tensioning versus knee stability. Knee Surg Sports Traumatol Arthrosc. 1998;6(Suppl 1):S38–42.
41. Odensten M, Gillquist J. Functional anatomy of the anterior cruciate ligament and a rationale for reconstruction. J Bone Joint Surg Am. 1985;67:257–62.
42. Odensten M, Gillquist J. A modified technique for anterior cruciate ligament surgery using a new drill guide for isometric positioning of the ACL. Clin Orthop Relat Res. 1986;213:154–8.
43. Bach BR Jr, Tradonsky S, Bojchuk J, Levy ME, Bush-Joseph CA, Khan NH (1998) Arthroscopically assisted anterior cruciate ligament reconstruction using patellar tendon autograft. Am J Sports Med 26:20–29.
44. Lewis PB, Parameswaran AD, Rue JP, Bach BR Jr. Systematic review of single-bundle anterior cruciate ligament reconstruction outcomes: a baseline assessment for consideration of double-bundle techniques. Am J Sports Med. 2008;36:2028–36.
45. Shen W, Jordan S, Fu F. Review article: anatomic double bundle anterior cruciate ligament reconstruction. J Orthop Surg (Hong Kong). 2007;15:216–21.
46. Aglietti P, Giron F, Cuomo P, Losco M, Mondanelli N. Single-and double-incision double-bundle ACL reconstruction. Clin Orthop Relat Res. 2007;454:108–13.

47. Järvelä T, Moisala A, Sihvonen R, Järvelä S, Kannus P, Järvinen M. Double-bundle anterior cruciate ligament reconstruction using hamstring autografts and bioabsorbable interference screw fixation. Am J Sports Med. 2008;36:290–8.
48. Fujie H, Mae T, Sekito T, Shino K. Mechanical functions of human ACL bundles: development and application of a robotic knee simulator. In: Kajzer J, Tanaka E, Yamada H, editors. Human biomechanics and injury prevention. Tokyo: Springer; 2000. p. 256–60.
49. Mae T, Shino K, Miyama T, Shinjo H, Ochi T, Yoshikawa H, Fujie H. Single- versus two-femoral socket anterior cruciate ligament reconstruction technique: biomechanical analysis using a robotic simulator. Arthroscopy. 2001;17:708–16.
50. Rosenberg TD, Brown GC, Deffner KT. Anterior cruciate ligament reconstruction with quadrupled semitendinosus autograft. Sports Med Arthrosc Rev. 1997;5:51–8.
51. Grood ES, Suntay WJ. A joint coordinate system for the clinical description three-dimensional motions: application to the knee. J Biomech Eng. 1983;105:136–44.
52. Butler DL, Guan Y, Kay MD, Cummings JF, Feder SM, Levy MS. Location-dependent variations in the material properties of the anterior cruciate ligament. J Biomech. 1992;25:511–8.
53. Scheffler SU, Maschewski K, Becker R, Asbach P. In-vivo three-dimensional MR imaging of the intact anterior cruciate ligament shows a variable insertion pattern of the femoral and tibial footprints. Knee Surg Sports Traumatol Arthrosc. 2018;26:3667–72.
54. Iriuchishima T, Ryu K, Aizawa S, Fu FH. Proportional evaluation of anterior cruciate ligament footprint size and knee bony morphology. Knee Surg Sports Traumatol Arthrosc. 2015;23:3157–62.
55. Morales-Avalos R, Perelli S, Vilchez-Cavazos F, Castillo-Escobedo T, Pena-Martinez VM, Elizondo-Omana R, et al. The morphology of the femoral footprint of the anterior cruciate ligament changes with aging from a large semi-circular shape to a small flat ribbon-like shape. Knee Surg Sports Traumatol Arthrosc. 2022;30:3402–13.
56. Smigielski R, Zdanowicz U, Drwiega M, Ciszek B, Ciszkowska-Lyson B, Siebold R. Ribbon like appearance of the midsubstance fibres of the anterior cruciate ligament close to its femoral insertion site: a cadaveric study including 111 knees. Knee Surg Sports Traumatol Arthrosc. 2015;23:3143–50.
57. Dimitriou D, Zou D, Wang Z, Helmy N, Tsai TY. Anterior cruciate ligament bundle insertions vary between ACL-rupture and non-injured knees. Knee Surg Sports Traumatol Arthrosc. 2021;29:1164–72.
58. Han Y, Kurzencwyg D, Hart A, Powell T, Martineau PA. Measuring the anterior cruciate ligament's footprints by three-dimensional magnetic resonance imaging. Knee Surg Sports Traumatol Arthrosc. 2012;20:986–95.
59. He M, Li J. Increased lateral femoral condyle ratio measured by MRI is associated with higher risk of noncontact anterior cruciate ligament injury. BMC Musculoskelet Disord. 2022;23:190.
60. Hodel S, Kabelitz M, Tondelli T, Vlachopoulos L, Sutter R, Fucentese SF. Introducing the Lateral Femoral Condyle Index as a risk factor for anterior cruciate ligament injury. Am J Sports Med. 2019;47:2420–6.
61. Shen L, Jin ZG, Dong QR, Li LB. Anatomical risk factors of anterior cruciate ligament injury. Chin Med J (Engl). 2018;131:2960–7.
62. Hart A, Sivakumaran T, Burman M, Powell T, Martineau PA. A prospective evaluation of femoral tunnel placement for anatomic anterior cruciate ligament reconstruction using 3-dimensional magnetic resonance imaging. Am J Sports Med. 2018;46:192–9.
63. Parkar AP, Adriaensen M, Vindfeld S, Solheim E. The anatomic centers of the femoral and tibial insertions of the anterior cruciate ligament: a systematic review of imaging and cadaveric studies reporting normal center locations. Am J Sports Med. 2017;45:2180–8.
64. Noailles T, Boisrenoult P, Sanchez M, Beaufils P, Pujol N. Torsional appearance of the anterior cruciate ligament explaining "ribbon" and double-bundle concepts: a cadaver-based study. Arthroscopy. 2017;33(9):1703–9.

65. Siebold R, Schuhmacher P, Fernandez F, Smigielski R, Brehmer A, Kirsch J. Flat midsubstance of the anterior cruciate ligament with tibial "C-"shaped insertion site. Knee Surg Sports Traumatol Arthrosc. 2015;23:3136–42.
66. Watanabe A, Kanamori A, Ikeda K, Ochiai N. Histological evaluation and comparison of the anteromedial and posterolateral bundle of the human anterior cruciate ligament of the osteoarthritic knee joint. Knee. 2011;18:47–50.
67. Tashiro Y, Lucidi GA, Gale T, Nagai K, Herbst E, Irrgang JJ, Nakashima Y, Anderst W, Fu FH. Anterior cruciate ligament tibial insertion site is elliptical or triangular shaped in healthy young adults: high-resolution 3-T MRI analysis. Knee Surg Sports Traumatol Arthrosc. 2018;26:485–90.
68. Fujimaki Y, Thorhauer E, Sasaki Y, Smolinski P, Tashman S, Fu FH. Quantitative in situ analysis of the anterior cruciate ligament: length, midsubstance cross-sectional area, and insertion site areas. Am J Sports Med. 2016;44(1):118–25.
69. Ferretti M, Levicoff EA, Macpherson TA, Moreland MS, Cohen M, Fu FH. The fetal anterior cruciate ligament: an anatomic and histologic study. Arthroscopy. 2007;23:278–83.
70. Tena-Arregui MD, Barrio-Asensio C, Viejo-Tirado F, Puerta-Fonolla J, Murilo-Gonzales J. Arthroscopic study of the knee joint in fetuses. Arthroscopy. 2003;19:862–8.
71. Driscoll MD, Isabell GP Jr, Conditt MA, Ismaily SK, Jupiter DC, Noble PC, Lowe WR. Comparison of 2 femoral tunnel locations in anatomic single-bundle anterior cruciate ligament reconstruction: a biomechanical study. Arthroscopy. 2012;28(10):1481–9.
72. Iriuchishima T, Ingham SJ, Tajima G, et al. Evaluation of the tunnel placement in the anatomical double-bundle ACL reconstruction: a cadaver study. Knee Surg Sports Traumatol Arthrosc. 2010;18(9):1226–31.
73. Maeyama A, Hoshino Y, Debandi A, et al. Evaluation of rotational instability in the anterior cruciate ligament deficient knee using triaxial accelerometer: a biomechanical model in porcine knees. Knee Surg Sports Traumatol Arthrosc. 2011;19(8):1233–8.
74. Siebold R, Ellert T, Metz S, Metz J. Femoral insertions of the anteromedial and posterolateral bundles of the anterior cruciate ligament: morphometry and arthroscopic orientation models for double-bundle bone tunnel placement—a cadaver study. Arthroscopy. 2008;24:585–92.
75. Woo SL, Hollis JM, Adams DJ, Lyon RM, Takai S. Tensile properties of the human femur-anterior cruciate ligamenttibia complex. The effects of specimen age and orientation. Am J Sports Med. 1991;19:217–25.
76. Iriuchishima T, Ryu K. A comparison of rollback ratio between bicruciate substituting total knee arthroplasty and Oxford unicompartmental knee arthroplasty. J Knee Surg. 2018;31(6):568–72.
77. Park YB, Ha CW, Kim HJ, Park YG. Preoperative prediction of anterior cruciate ligament tibial footprint size by anthropometric variables. Knee Surg Sports Traumatol Arthrosc. 2017;25(5):1638–45.
78. Wu E, Chen M, Cooperman D, Victoroff B, Goodfellow D, Farrow LD. No correlation of height or gender with anterior cruciate ligament footprint size. J Knee Surg. 2011;24:39–43.
79. Cha PS, Brucker PU, West RV, Zelle BA, Yagi M, Kurosaka M, Fu FH. Arthroscopic double-bundle anterior cruciate ligament reconstruction: an anatomic approach. Arthroscopy. 2005;21:1275.
80. Forster MC, Forster IW. Patellar tendon or four-strand hamstring? A systematic review of autografts for anterior cruciate ligament reconstruction. Knee. 2005;12:225–30.
81. Chen WT, Shih TT, Tu HY, Chen RC, Shau WY. Partial and complete tear of the anterior cruciate ligament. Acta Radiol. 2002;43:511–6.
82. Kocabey Y, Tetik O, Isbell WM, Atay OA, Johnson DL. The value of clinical examination versus magnetic resonance imaging in the diagnosis of meniscal tears and anterior cruciate ligament rupture. Arthroscopy. 2004;20:696–700.
83. Tsai KJ, Chiang H, Jiang CC. Magnetic resonance imaging of anterior cruciate ligament rupture. BMC Musculoskelet Disord. 2004;5:21.

84. Duc SR, Zanetti M, Kramer J, Kach KP, Zollikofer CL, Wentz KU. MRI of anterior cruciate ligament tears: evaluation of standard orthogonal and tailored paracoronal images. Acta Radiol. 2005;46:729–33.
85. Lawrance JA, Ostlere SJ, Dodd CA. MRI diagnosis of partial tears of the anterior cruciate ligament. Injury. 1996;27:153–5.
86. McCauley TR, Moses M, Kier R, Lynch JK, Barton JW, Jokl P. MR diagnosis of tears of anterior cruciate ligament of the knee: importance of ancillary findings. AJR Am J Roentgenol. 1994;162:115–9.
87. Roychowdhury S, Fitzgerald SW, Sonin AH, Peduto AJ, Miller FH, Hoff FL. Using MR imaging to diagnose partial tears of the anterior cruciate ligament: value of axial images. Am J Roentgenol. 1997;168:1487–91.
88. Tung GA, Davis LM, Wiggins ME, Fadale PD. Tears of the anterior cruciate ligament: primary and secondary signs at MR imaging. Radiology. 1993;188:661–7.
89. Umans H, Wimpfheimer O, Haramati N, Applbaum YH, Adler M, Bosco J. Diagnosis of partial tears of the anterior cruciate ligament of the knee: value of MR imaging. Am J Roentgenol. 1995;165:893–7.
90. Mellado JM, Calmet J, Olona M, Gine J, Sauri A. Magnetic resonance imaging of anterior cruciate ligament tears: reevaluation of quantitative parameters and imaging findings including a simplified method for measuring the anterior cruciate ligament angle. Knee Surg Sports Traumatolo Arthrosc. 2004;12:217–24.
91. Amis AA, Dawkins GP. Functional anatomy of the anterior cruciate ligament. Fibre bundle actions related to ligament replacements and injuries. J Bone Joint Surg Br. 1991;73:260–7.
92. Duthon VB, Barea C, Abrassart S, Fasel JH, Fritschy D, Ménétrey J. Anatomy of the anterior cruciate ligament. Knee Surg Sports Traumatol Arthrosc. 2005; https://doi.org/10.1007/s00167-005-0679-9.
93. Bicer EK, Lustig S, Servien E, Selmi TAS, Neyret P. Current knowledge in the anatomy of the human anterior cruciate ligament. Knee Surg Sports Traumatol Arthrosc. 2009; https://doi.org/10.1007/s00167-009-0993-8.
94. Fujie H, Otsubo H, Fukano S, Suzuki T, Suzuki D, Mae T, Shino K. Mechanical functions of the three bundles consisting of the human anterior cruciate ligament. Knee Surg Sports Traumatol Arthrosc. 2011; https://doi.org/10.1007/s00167-011-1513-1.
95. Lin J, Zhang S, Xin E, Liang M, Yang L, Chen J. Anterior cruciate ligament femoral footprint is oblong-ovate, triangular, or two-tears shaped in healthy young adults: three-dimensional MRI analysis. Knee Surg Sports Traumatol Arthrosc. 2023; https://doi.org/10.1007/s00167-023-07606-6.
96. Morales-Avalos R, Castillo-Escobedo TA, Elizondo-Omaña RE, del Carmen Theriot-Giron M, Perelli S, Guzmán-López S, Peña-Martínez VM, Vílchez-Cavazos F, Monllau JC. The morphology of the tibial footprint of the anterior cruciate ligament changes with ageing from oval/elliptical to C-shaped. Knee Surg Sports Traumatol Arthrosc. 2020; https://doi.org/10.1007/s00167-020-06049-7.
97. Iriuchishima T, Ryu K, Fu FH. Evaluation of age-related differences in anterior cruciate ligament size. Knee Surg Sports Traumatol Arthrosc. 2018; https://doi.org/10.1007/s00167-018-5336-1.
98. Steckel H, Vadala G, Davis D, Fu FH. 2D and 3D 3-tesla magnetic resonance imaging of the double bundle structure in anterior cruciate ligament anatomy. Knee Surg Sports Traumatol Arthrosc. 2006; https://doi.org/10.1007/s00167-006-0185-8.

Chapter 2
Posterior Cruciate Ligament and Related Ligaments

Alfred J. Tria Jr. and Giles R. Scuderi

Introduction by the Editor

The posterior cruciate ligament (PCL) is a central stabilizer of the knee that prevents posterior motion in both full extension and 90 degrees of flexion. It is embryologically present by 6 weeks of gestation [5]. The ligament is composed of 2 bundles (with one article suggesting that there are 3). Its blood supply is from the middle geniculate. Scapinelli confirmed this with his autopsy dissections and contrast injections. There is minimal supply from the bone origin or insertion [55]. Schutte et al. identified mechanoreceptors and free nerve endings that account for motion, speed, acceleration, and pain reception. The innervations account for proprioception [56]. The double bundle structure enables the ligament to stabilize the knee throughout the range of motion [41].

Machine Generated Summaries

Disclaimer: The summaries in this chapter were generated from Springer Nature publications using abstractive AI auto-summarization: An abstraction-based summarizer creates new text based on deep learning. New phrases are created to summarize the content. As the constituted sentences are machine selected, they may not fully reflect the body of the work, so we strongly advise that the original content is

A. J. Tria Jr. (✉)
Department of Orthopedics, Rutgers-Robert Wood Johnson Medical School, New Brunswick, NJ, USA

G. R. Scuderi
Northwell Health Orthopaedic Institute, New York, NY, USA

A. J. Tria Jr., G. R. Scuderi (eds.), *Ligaments of the Knee*,
https://doi.org/10.1007/978-3-031-66615-5_2

read and cited. The auto-generated summaries were curated by the editor to meet Springer Nature publication standards.

Machine generated keywords: reconstruction, mfls, pcl reconstruction, preserve, mfl, technique, footprint, pcl, tibial, patient, remnant, remnant preserve, dimple, posterior dimple, variant.

Posterior Cruciate Ligament: Anatomy and Biomechanics [49]

This is a machine-generated summary of:

Logterman, Stephanie L.; Wydra, Frank B.; Frank, Rachel M.: Posterior Cruciate Ligament: Anatomy and Biomechanics [49]

Published in: Current Reviews in Musculoskeletal Medicine (2018)

Link to original: https://doi.org/10.1007/s12178-018-9492-1

If you want to cite the papers, please refer to the original.

For technical reasons we could not place the page where the original quote is coming from.

Research Highlights

The posterior cruciate ligament (PCL) is a key stabilizer in the knee, essential for maintaining proper kinematics and load distribution during movement. Despite its importance, PCL injuries are less common than those to the anterior cruciate ligament (ACL), leading to a relative paucity of research on its complex anatomy and biomechanics. A study by Logterman et al. provides a review of the most recent literature on PCL anatomy and biomechanics, offering valuable insights for physicians in the evaluation, diagnosis, and treatment of PCL injuries.

Logterman compiled data from various cadaveric, imaging, and arthroscopic studies to map out the details of the PCL's structure. The research delves into the characteristics of the PCL's two functional bundles—the anterolateral bundle (ALB) and posteromedial bundle (PMB)—and their respective attachment sites on the femur and tibia. The study also examines surrounding structures within the knee, such as the popliteal artery and vein, which are critical considerations during surgical procedures. By integrating findings from multiple studies, including those that measure distances between key anatomical landmarks and explore the impact of knee flexion angles on ligament tensioning, Logterman et al. have synthesized a comprehensive guide to PCL anatomy that is poised to enhance surgical precision.

The main advance presented by Logterman is a detailed understanding of how the PCL's two bundles contribute to knee stability through their distinct tensioning patterns across different ranges of motion. This knowledge is crucial for reconstructing the ligament anatomically and with appropriate tension to restore native knee function. As Logterman suggests, while current knowledge about the PCL is extensive, there remains a need for further research into the nuances of its biomechanics to optimize patient outcomes following injury. The study not only reinforces the complexity of PCL anatomy but also underscores its significance in maintaining knee stability—a foundation upon which future research can build more targeted therapeutic strategies.

Bony Landmark Between the Attachment of the Medial Meniscus Posterior Root and the Posterior Cruciate Ligament: Ct and MR Imaging Assessment [50]

This is a machine-generated summary of:

Fujii, Masataka; Furumatsu, Takayuki; Miyazawa, Shinichi; Kodama, Yuya; Hino, Tomohito; Kamatsuki, Yusuke; Ozaki, Toshifumi: Bony landmark between the attachment of the medial meniscus posterior root and the posterior cruciate ligament: CT and MR imaging assessment [50]

Published in: Skeletal Radiology (2017)

Link to original: https://doi.org/10.1007/s00256-017-2625-6

If you want to cite the papers, please refer to the original.

For technical reasons we could not place the page where the original quote is coming from.

Research Highlights

The integrity of the medial meniscus, particularly its posterior root attachment, is crucial for preserving knee joint cartilage and preventing osteoarthritis. Despite advancements in meniscal root repair surgery, such as transosseous pullout repair, challenges remain in accurately positioning the tibial tunnel due to the complex anatomy of the knee and potential neurovascular risks associated with advanced arthroscopic techniques. Fujii et al. address this issue by investigating a novel anatomical landmark, termed the "posterior dimple," which could aid in evaluating tunnel position during ligament reconstruction or meniscal root repair surgeries.

Fujii utilized three-dimensional computed tomography (CT) and magnetic resonance imaging (MRI) to analyze the position of the posterior dimple relative to other critical structures within the knee. The study was conducted following IRB approval and informed consent from patients who had undergone anterior cruciate ligament (ACL) reconstructions. The team employed advanced imaging techniques and software for precise measurements, ensuring high inter- and intra-observer reliability. Fujii suggested that the posterior dimple is a consistent anatomical feature that could serve as a reliable landmark for surgeons.

The study revealed that the posterior dimple was present in a significant percentage of knees and consistently located between the tibial attachment of the posterior cruciate ligament (PCL) and the medial meniscus posterior root insertion (MMPI). This discovery offers surgeons a new reference point for improving surgical outcomes. The identification of this bony recess could revolutionize tibial tunnel placement in PCL reconstruction.

The main advance from this study is the identification of the posterior dimple as a potential anatomical landmark for more accurate tibial tunnel positioning in PCL reconstruction and medial meniscal root repair surgeries. This could lead to improved surgical precision and potentially better patient outcomes. While acknowledging limitations such as sample diversity and visibility during arthroscopy, Fujii suggests future research is needed across diverse populations and additional histological analysis are needed to fully understand the implications of this landmark. These observations paves the way for enhancing surgical techniques that could mitigate complications associated with current methods.

Successful Reconstruction of the Posterior Cruciate Ligament: Assessment of Posterior Cruciate Ligament Footprints Using an Objective Coordinate System [51]

This is a machine-generated summary of:

Vielgut, Ines; Weiglein, Andreas; Biber, Stefan M.; Dreu, Manuel; Leithner, Andreas; Hohenberger, Goria; Sadoghi, Patrick: Successful reconstruction of the posterior cruciate ligament: assessment of posterior cruciate ligament footprints using an objective coordinate system [51]

Published in: Surgical and Radiologic Anatomy (2020)

Link to original: https://doi.org/10.1007/s00276-020-02520-9

If you want to cite the papers, please refer to the original.

For technical reasons we could not place the page where the original quote is coming from.

Research Highlights

Injuries to the posterior cruciate ligament (PCL) are significant yet often underdiagnosed, leading to knee instability and long-term complications such as osteoarthritis. Traditional reconstruction techniques have aimed for isometry, assuming a fixed ligament length throughout the knee's range of motion, but this has led to joint over-constraint and increased laxity over time. Ines Vielgut et al. address the need for precise anatomical knowledge in PCL reconstruction by providing detailed measurements of the ligament's tibial and femoral insertion sites.

Vielgut conducted an anatomical study on donated bodies, employing Thiel's preservation technique to maintain tissue pliability. After transecting associated ligaments for clear access, they meticulously identified and marked the PCL insertion points. Utilizing a coordinate system based on anatomical landmarks, they captured standardized photographs from specific angles to ensure accurate representation of the insertion sites. Vielgut performed measurements twice within a two-week interval to assess reproducibility using Cohen's kappa coefficient. Their methodology offers a promising approach to improving surgical outcomes by enabling more precise preoperative planning and potentially informing the development of custom surgical tools.

The study's findings underscore the potential for enhanced surgical techniques in PCL reconstruction. Vielgut 's method demonstrates high repeatability and reproducibility, suggesting that their precise mapping of PCL insertion sites could significantly improve graft placement accuracy during surgery. This advancement may lead to better restoration of knee stability and function post-reconstruction. Looking forward, these insights could pave the way for integrating three-dimensional imaging with the team's coordinate system to further refine surgical planning. While acknowledging limitations such as not distinguishing between anterolateral and posteromedial bundle insertion sites, Vielgut emphasizes the benefits of their standardized approach across a large sample size, setting a new benchmark for anatomical studies in PCL reconstruction.

Posterior Cruciate Ligament Is Twisted and Flat Structure: New Prospective on Anatomical Morphology [52]

This is a machine-generated summary of:

Kato, Tomohiro; Śmigielski, Robert; Ge, Yunshen; Zdanowicz, Urszula; Ciszek, Bogdan; Ochi, Mitsuo: Posterior cruciate ligament is twisted and flat structure: new prospective on anatomical morphology [52]

Published in: Knee Surgery, Sports Traumatology, Arthroscopy (2017)

Link to original: https://doi.org/10.1007/s00167-017-4634-3

If you want to cite the papers, please refer to the original.

For technical reasons we could not place the page where the original quote is coming from.

Research Highlights

Injuries to the posterior cruciate ligament (PCL) are a common affliction among athletes engaged in contact sports, with isolated PCL injuries traditionally managed through conservative treatment. Although this approach often yields satisfactory results, some patients experience residual instability. Kato et al. elucidate the detailed morphology of the PCL and its associated structures using fresh-frozen cadaveric knees, with a focus on optimizing remnant preserving PCL reconstruction techniques.

The authors dissected 17 unpaired cadaveric knees, adhering to ethical standards for human cadaver research in Poland. They removed surrounding soft tissues to expose the PCL, ligaments of Humphrey and Wrisberg, and then conducted precise measurements of these structures. The goal was to understand the intricate anatomy that is crucial for successful surgical outcomes,. The researchers employed various methods such as digital photography, vernier calipers for direct measurements, and ImageJ software for cross-sectional area calculations. They also utilized the clock-face method to understand the anatomical positioning within the knee joint. Through this comprehensive analysis, Kato uncovered that the PCL at midsubstance is flat with a twisted ribbon-like structure, challenging traditional notions of distinct PCL bundles.

The study's main advance lies in its detailed characterization of the PCL's morphology and its relationship with adjacent ligaments. Kato noted that their findings have significant implications for remnant preserving PCL reconstruction. By revealing that the PCL comprises interconnected fibers rather than separate bundles, surgeons can better appreciate the complexity of this ligament during reconstructive procedures. Looking forward, these insights could influence both the surgical approach to PCL injuries and the design of grafts used in reconstruction, potentially improving patient outcomes after surgery.

Evaluation of Age-Dependent Morphometrics of the Meniscofemoral Ligaments in Reference to the Posterior Cruciate Ligament in Routine MRI [53]

This is a machine-generated summary of:

Röhrich, Sebastian; Kainberger, Franz; Hirtler, Lena: Evaluation of age-dependent morphometrics of the meniscofemoral ligaments in reference to the posterior cruciate ligament in routine MRI [53]

Published in: European Radiology (2018)

Link to original: https://doi.org/10.1007/s00330-017-5128-x

If you want to cite the papers, please refer to the original.

For technical reasons we could not place the page where the original quote is coming from.

Research Highlights

The anterior and posterior meniscofemoral ligaments (MFLs) play a crucial role in knee joint stability, yet their morphological characteristics remain inconsistently reported, leading to a knowledge gap in standardizing their identification, particularly in magnetic resonance imaging (MRI). Age-related changes further complicate the understanding of MFL morphology and function. Röhrich et al. address this gap by quantifying the morphological relationship between the posterior cruciate ligament (PCL) and MFLs across different age groups, proposing MRI identification guidelines to aid in accurate diagnosis and treatment planning.

Röhrich's cross-sectional retrospective study analyzed knee MRIs from a diverse patient cohort, stratified into five age groups. The researchers employed a standardized protocol on a 3-Tesla MRI scanner to measure variables such as the presence, length, running angle, and cross-sectional area (CSA) of the MFLs. Two experienced musculoskeletal radiologists independently reviewed the images to ensure robust inter-rater reliability. The study revealed no statistical significant gender differences in MFL presence, but did uncover significant age-related variations in MFL morphology.

The findings highlight that at least one MFL was present in the majority of cases, with the CSA of the PCL being larger when the pMFL was absent, suggesting compensatory thickening. Interestingly, single MFLs exhibited larger CSAs than when both were present, indicating a potential adaptive mechanism. These results underscore the dynamic nature of knee ligament morphology across the lifespan.

By establishing normal ranges for MFLs from childhood to old age and proposing MRI identification guidelines, this study provides valuable insights for orthopedic surgeons and radiologists. The authors suggest that future research should explore longitudinal changes in MFL morphology and its implications for knee pathology development. This work not only refines diagnostic accuracy but also has potential implications for surgical planning and patient outcomes in ligamentous injuries of the knee.

A Novel Meniscofemoral Ligament Variant Intra-Substance to the PCL [54]

This is a machine-generated summary of:

Verhey, Jens T.; Deckey, David G.; Tummala, Sailesh; Hassebrock, Jeffrey D.; Dulle, Donald; Long, Jeremiah R.; Miller, Mark D.; Chhabra, Anikar: A novel meniscofemoral ligament variant intra-substance to the PCL [54]

Published in: Knee Surgery, Sports Traumatology, Arthroscopy (2021)

Link to original: https://doi.org/10.1007/s00167-021-06791-6

If you want to cite the papers, please refer to the original.

For technical reasons we could not place the page where the original quote is coming from.

Research Highlights

Knee injuries are a common occurrence, often leading to chronic pain and instability that can significantly impact a patient's quality of life. Despite advances in imaging and surgical techniques, there remains a knowledge gap in the full understanding of knee joint anatomy, particularly concerning less common anatomical variants that may influence injury patterns and treatment outcomes. Verhey et al. identified a novel anatomical variant of the meniscofemoral ligament (MFL) within the posterior cruciate ligament (PCL), which they propose to name the internal meniscofemoral ligament (iMFL).

The investigation included physical examination, imaging, and surgical intervention to explore the patient's persistent knee issues. The MRI scans revealed not only meniscal tears and chondromalacia but also an unusual ligamentous variant through the PCL—a previously undocumented iMFL. During surgery, this variant was meticulously visualized, confirming its unique pathway through the PCL and its distinct origin from other known MFLs. The authors suggest that this iMFL could play a role in knee stability and may be implicated in injury mechanisms. The study combined advanced imaging with detailed arthroscopic examination, providing a comprehensive analysis of this anatomical anomaly.

The discovery of the iMFL represents a significant advance in our understanding of knee joint anatomy and its potential implications for injury risk and surgical treatment. Verhey's findings suggest that the presence of this ligament variant may predispose patients to specific injury patterns, particularly involving the PCL. Looking forward, the authors emphasize the importance of recognizing such anatomical variations during arthroscopy to tailor surgical interventions more effectively. Future investigations on MFL variants may guide surgical management of PCL and meniscal root injuries. This research paves the way for further studies into the biomechanical functions of MFLs and their impact on knee stability, which could ultimately lead to improved outcomes for patients with complex knee injuries.

Bibliography

1. Anderson CJ, Ziegler CG, Wijdicks CA, Engebretsen L, LaPrade RF. Arthroscopically pertinent anatomy of the anterolateral and posteromedial bundles of the posterior cruciate ligament. J Bone Joint Surg Am. 2012;94(21):1936–45. https://doi.org/10.2106/JBJS.K.01710. This reference is important as it nicely shows the arthroscopic anatomy of the PCL, which is helpful for surgeons performing PCL reconstruction.
2. LaPrade CM, Civitarese DM, Rasmussen MT, LaPrade RF. Emerging updates on the posterior cruciate ligament: a review of the current literature. Am J Sports Med. 2015; https://doi.org/10.1177/0363546515572770.
3. Girgis FG, Marshall JL, Monajem A. The cruciate ligaments of the knee joint. Anatomical, functional and experimental analysis. Clin Orthop Relat Res. 1975;106(106):216–31.
4. Van Dommelen BA, Fowler PJ. Anatomy of the posterior cruciate ligament: a review. Am J Sports Med. 1989;17(1):24–9. https://doi.org/10.1177/036354658901700104.
5. Harner CD, Janaushek MA, Kanamori A, Yagi M, Vogrin TM, Woo SL. Biomechanical analysis of a double-bundle posterior cruciate ligament reconstruction. Am J Sports Med. 2000;28(2):144–51. http://www.ncbi.nlm.nih.gov/pubmed/10750988
6. Kennedy NI, LaPrade RF, Goldsmith MT, et al. Posterior cruciate ligament graft fixation angles, part 1: biomechanical evaluation for anatomic single-bundle reconstruction. https://doi.org/10.1177/0363546514541225.
7. Gollehon DL, Torzilli PA, Warren RF. The role of the posterolateral and cruciate ligaments in the stability of the human knee. A biomechanical study. J Bone Joint Surg Am. 1987;69(2):233–42. https://doi.org/10.1177/036354659502300411.
8. Grood ES, Stowers SF, Noyes FR. Limits of movement in the human knee. Effect of sectioning the posterior cruciate ligament and posterolateral structures. J Bone Joint Surg Am. 1988;70(1):88–97.
9. Marzo JM, Gurske-DePerio J. Effects of medial meniscus posterior horn avulsion and repair on tibiofemoral contact area and peak contact pressure with clinical implications. Am J Sports Med. 2009;37(1):124–9.
10. Chung KS, Ha JK, Ra HJ, Nam GW, Kim JG. Pullout fixation of posterior medial meniscus root tears: correlation between meniscus extrusion and midterm clinical results. Am J Sports Med. 2016.
11. Lavender CD, Hanzlik SR, Caldwell PE 3rd, Pearson SE. Transosseous medial meniscal root repair using a modified Mason-Allen suture configuration. Arthrosc Tech. 2015;4(6):e781–4.
12. LaPrade RF, Matheny LM, Moulton SG, James EW, Dean CS. Posterior meniscal root repairs: outcomes of an anatomic transtibial pull-out technique. Am J Sports Med. 2016.
13. Harner CD, Baek GH, Vogrin TM, Carlin GJ, Kashiwaguchi S, Woo SL. Quantitative analysis of human cruciate ligament insertions. Arthroscopy. 1999;15(7):741–9. https://doi.org/10.1016/S0749-8063(99)70006-X.
14. Voos JE, Md Y, Mauro CS, Wente T, Warren RF, Wickiewicz TL. Posterior cruciate ligament anatomy, biomechanics, and outcomes. https://doi.org/10.1177/0363546511416316.
15. Urban WP Jr, Nyland J, Caborn DN, Johnson DL. The radiographic position of medial and lateral meniscal horns as a basis for meniscal reconstruction. Arthroscopy. 1999;15(2):147–54.
16. Kodama Y, Furumatsu T, Miyazawa S, Fujii M, Tanaka T, Inoue H, Ozaki T. Location of the tibial tunnel aperture affects extrusion of the lateral meniscus following reconstruction of the anterior cruciate ligament. J Orthop Res. 2016; https://doi.org/10.1002/jor.23450.

17. Kim SJ, Jung M, Moon HK, Kim SG, Chun YM. Anterolateral transtibial posterior cruciate ligament reconstruction combined with anatomical reconstruction of posterolateral corner insufficiency: comparison of single-bundle versus double-bundle posterior cruciate ligament reconstruction over a 2- to 6-year follow-up. Am J Sports Med. 2011;39(3):481–9.
18. Kim YK, Yoo JD, Kim SW, Park SH, Cho JH, Lim HM. Intraoperative graft isometry in anatomic single-bundle anterior cruciate ligament reconstruction. Knee Surg Relat Res. 2018;30(2):115–20.
19. Ahn JH, Yang HS, Jeong WK, Koh KH. Arthroscopic transtibial posterior cruciate ligament reconstruction with preservation of posterior cruciate ligament fibers: clinical results of minimum 2-year follow-up. Am J Sports Med. 2006;34(2):194–204.
20. Dargel J, Pohl P, Tzikaras P, Koebke J. Morphometric side-to-side differences in human cruciate ligament insertions. Surg Radiol Anat. 2006;28(4):398–402.
21. Del Buono A, Radmilovic J, Gargano G, Gatto S, Maffulli N. Augmentation or reconstruction of PCL? A quantitative review. Knee Surg Sports Traumatol Arthrosc. 2006;21(5):1050–63.
22. Lee KH, et al. Combined posterolateral corner reconstruction with remnant tensioning and augmentation in chronic posterior cruciate ligament injuries: minimum 2-year follow-up. Arthroscopy. 2011;27(4):507–15.
23. Nuelle CW, et al. Biomechanical comparison of five posterior cruciate ligament reconstruction techniques. J Knee Surg. 2017;30(4):347–51.
24. Orakzai SH, Egan CM, Eustace S, Kenny P, O'Flanagan SJ, Keogh P. Correlation of intra-articular osseous measurements with posterior cruciate ligament length on MRI scans. Br J Radiol. 2010;83(985):23–7.
25. Naraghi A, White LM. MR imaging of cruciate ligaments. Magn Reson Imaging Clin N Am. 2014;22(4):557–80.
26. Sadoghi P, et al. Evaluating the tibial and femoral insertion site of the anterior cruciate ligament using an objective coordinate system: a cadaver study. Injury. 2012;43:1771–5.
27. Milles JL, et al. Biomechanical comparison: single-bundle versus double-bundle posterior cruciate ligament reconstruction techniques. J Knee Surg. 2017;30(4):347–51.
28. Schmeiser G, Hempfling H, Bühren V, Putz R. The popliteal region: an anatomical study and a new approach to the tibial attachment of the posterior cruciate ligament. Surg Radiol Anat. 2001;23(1):9–14.
29. Shin YS, Kim HJ, Lee DH. No clinically important difference in knee scores or instability between transtibial and inlay techniques for PCL reconstruction: a systematic review. Clin Orthop Relat Res. 2017;475:1239.
30. Johannsen AM, Anderson CJ, Wijdicks CA, Engebretsen L, LaPrade RF. Radiographic landmarks for tunnel positioning in posterior cruciate ligament reconstructions. Am J Sports Med. 2013; https://doi.org/10.1177/0363546512465072.
31. Race A, Amis AA. PCL reconstruction: in vitro biomechanical comparison of "isometric" versus single and double-bundled "anatomic" grafts. J Bone Joint Surg Br. 1998;80(1):173–9.
32. Sadoghi P, Kropfl A, Jansson V, Müller PE, Pietschmann MF, Fischmeister MF. Impact of tibial and femoral tunnel position on clinical results after anterior cruciate ligament reconstruction. Arthroscopy. 2011;27(3):355–64.
33. Teng Y, Guo L, Wu M, Xu T, Zhao L, Jiang J, Sheng X, Xu L, Zhang B, Ding N, Xia Y. MRI analysis of tibial PCL attachment in a large population of adult patients: reference data for anatomic PCL reconstruction. BMC Musculoskelet Disord. 2016;17(1):384.
34. Adachi N, Ochi M, Uchio Y, Iwasa J, Ishikawa M, Shinomiya R. Temporal change of joint position sense after posterior cruciate ligament reconstruction using multi-stranded hamstring tendons. Knee Surg Sports Traumatol Arthrosc. 2007;15(1):2–8.
35. Ahn JH, Chung YS, Oh I. Arthroscopic posterior cruciate ligament reconstruction using the posterior trans-septal portal. Arthroscopy. 2003;19(1):101–7.
36. Ahn JH, Lee SH. Anatomic graft passage in remnant-preserving posterior cruciate ligament reconstruction. Arthrosc Tech. 2014;3(5):e579–82.

37. Ahn JH, Nha KW, Kim YC, Lim HC, Nam HW, Wang JH. Arthroscopic femoral tensioning and posterior cruciate ligament reconstruction in chronic posterior cruciate ligament injury. Arthroscopy. 2006;22(3):e341–4.
38. Eguchi A, Adachi N, Nakamae A, Usman MA, Deie M, Ochi M. Proprioceptive function after isolated single-bundle posterior cruciate ligament reconstruction with remnant preservation for chronic posterior cruciate ligament injuries. Orthop Traumatol Surg Res. 2014;100(3):303–8.
39. Jung HJ, Kim JH, Lee HJ, Koo S, Chang SH, Jung YB, Lee SH. The isometry of two different paths for remnant-preserving posterior cruciate ligament reconstruction. Knee Surg Sports Traumatol Arthrosc. 2013;5:1029–35.
40. Lee DW, Jang HW, Lee YS, Oh SJ, Kim JY, Song HE, Kim JG. Clinical, functional, and morphological evaluations of posterior cruciate ligament reconstruction with remnant preservation: minimum 2-year follow-up. Am J Sports Med. 2014;42(8):1822–31.
41. Amis AA, Gupte CM, Bull AM, Edwards A. Anatomy of the posterior cruciate ligament and the meniscofemoral ligaments. Knee Surg Sports Traumatol Arthrosc. 2006;14(3):257–63.
42. Gupte CM, Smith A, McDermott ID, Bull AM, Thomas RD, Amis AA. Meniscofemoral ligaments revisited. Anatomical study, age correlation and clinical implications. J Bone Joint Surg. 2002;84:846–51.
43. Bintoudi A, Natsis K, Tsitouridis I. Anterior and posterior meniscofemoral ligaments: MRI evaluation. Anat Res Int. 2012;2012:839724.
44. Forkel P, Reuter S, Sprenker F, et al. Different patterns of lateral meniscus root tears in ACL injuries: application of a differentiated classification system. Knee Surg Sports Traumatol Arthrosc: Official J ESSKA. 2015;23:112–8.
45. Gupte CM, Bull AM, Thomas RD, Amis AA. A review of the function and biomechanics of the meniscofemoral ligaments. Arthrosc Assoc North Am Int Arthrosc Assoc. 2003;19:161–71.
46. Woo SL, Hollis JM, Adams DJ, Lyon RM, Takai S. Tensile properties of the human femur-anterior cruciate ligament-tibia complex. The effects of specimen age and orientation. Am J Sports Med. 1991;19:217–25.
47. Arthur JR, Haglin JM, Makovicka JL, Chhabra A. Anatomy and biomechanics of the posterior cruciate ligament and their surgical implications. Sports Med Arthrosc Rev. 2020;28:e1–e10.
48. Gupte CM, Shaerf DA, Sandison A, Bull AM, Amis AA. Neural structures within human meniscofemoral ligaments: a cadaveric study. ISRN Anat. 2014;2014:719851.
49. Logterman SL, Wydra FB, Frank RM. Posterior cruciate ligament: anatomy and biomechanics. Curr Rev Musculoskelet Med. 2018; https://doi.org/10.1007/s12178-018-9492-1.
50. Fujii M, Furumatsu T, Miyazawa S, Kodama Y, Hino T, Kamatsuki Y, Ozaki T. Bony landmark between the attachment of the medial meniscus posterior root and the posterior cruciate ligament: CT and MR imaging assessment. Skeletal Radiol. 2017; https://doi.org/10.1007/s00256-017-2625-6.
51. Vielgut I, Weiglein A, Biber SM, Dreu M, Leithner A, Hohenberger G, Sadoghi P. Successful reconstruction of the posterior cruciate ligament: assessment of posterior cruciate ligament footprints using an objective coordinate system. Surg Radiol Anat. 2020; https://doi.org/10.1007/s00276-020-02520-9.
52. Kato T, Śmigielski R, Ge Y, Zdanowicz U, Ciszek B, Ochi M. Posterior cruciate ligament is twisted and flat structure: new prospective on anatomical morphology. Knee Surg Sports Traumatol Arthrosc. 2017; https://doi.org/10.1007/s00167-017-4634-3.
53. Röhrich S, Kainberger F, Hirtler L. Evaluation of age-dependent morphometrics of the meniscofemoral ligaments in reference to the posterior cruciate ligament in routine MRI. Eur Radiol. 2018; https://doi.org/10.1007/s00330-017-5128-x.
54. Verhey JT, Deckey DG, Tummala S, Hassebrock JD, Dulle D, Long JR, Miller MD, Chhabra A. A novel meniscofemoral ligament variant intra-substance to the PCL. Knee Surg Sports Traumatol Arthrosc. 2021; https://doi.org/10.1007/s00167-021-06791-6.

55. Scapinelli R. Vascular anatomy of the human cruciate ligaments and surrounding structures. Clin Anat. 1997;10:151–62.
56. Schutte MJ, Dabezies EJ, Zimny ML, Happel LT. Neural anatomy of the human anterior cruciate ligament. J Bone Joint Surg Am. 1987;69:243–7.

Chapter 3
The Medial Collateral Ligament and Posteromedial Ligament Complex

Alfred J. Tria Jr. and Giles R. Scuderi

Introduction by the Editor

The medial collateral ligament is the primary stabilizer of the knee to valgus stress. The deep and superficial portions have been thoroughly studied and further evaluations have contributed to greater understanding and more refined surgical approaches.

Machine Generated Summaries

Disclaimer: The summaries in this chapter were generated from Springer Nature publications using abstractive AI auto-summarization: An abstraction-based summarizer creates new text based on deep learning. New phrases are created to summarize the content. As the constituted sentences are machine selected, they may not fully reflect the body of the work, so we strongly advise that the original content is read and cited. The auto-generated summaries were curated by the editor to meet Springer Nature publication standards.

Machine generated keywords: fascia, mcl, pol, tendon, injury, posterior, insertion, joint, paratenon, band, accessory, capsule, joint capsule, mme, accessory band.

A. J. Tria Jr. (✉)
Department of Orthopedics, Rutgers-Robert Wood Johnson Medical School, New Brunswick, NJ, USA

G. R. Scuderi
Northwell Health Orthopaedic Institute, New York, NY, USA

A. J. Tria Jr., G. R. Scuderi (eds.), *Ligaments of the Knee*,
https://doi.org/10.1007/978-3-031-66615-5_3

Morphology of the Medial Collateral Ligament of the Knee [52]

This is a machine-generated summary of:

Liu, Fang; Yue, Bing; Gadikota, Hemanth R; Kozanek, Michal; Liu, Wanjun; Gill, Thomas J; Rubash, Harry E; Li, Guoan: Morphology of the medial collateral ligament of the knee [52]

Published in: Journal of Orthopaedic Surgery and Research (2010)

Link to original: https://doi.org/10.1186/1749-799x-5-69

If you want to cite the papers, please refer to the original.

For technical reasons we could not place the page where the original quote is coming from.

Research Highlights

The medial collateral ligament (MCL) is a critical structure in maintaining knee stability, particularly against valgus forces. In total knee arthroplasty (TKA), achieving proper knee alignment often necessitates partial release of the MCL, making a comprehensive understanding of its anatomy essential for surgical success. Despite numerous studies on the MCL, discrepancies exist regarding the precise femoral attachment of the superficial MCL (sMCL), and data on the deep MCL (dMCL) remains sparse. Liu et al. addressed this by quantitatively dissecting the morphology of the MCL in human cadaveric knees.

Liu dissected ten cadaveric knees to map out the sMCL and dMCL's insertion sites, lengths, and their relationships to key anatomical landmarks. Utilizing a digitizing system with high accuracy, the researchers transferred these physical measurements into a solid modeling software to calculate precise areas and centroids. They found that while the sMCL is triangular and firmly attached to the medial meniscus posteriorly, the dMCL is thinner and has distinct femoral and tibial insertion areas. Their methodical approach involved separating the sMCL from the dMCL without damage, detaching pes anserinus tendons for clear visualization, and using statistical analysis to compare various dimensions of these ligaments.

The findings offer significant advances in our understanding of MCL anatomy. It provides detailed quantitative data on both sMCL and dMCL components, which had not been statistically compared before. The research confirms some previous assumptions about sMCL attachments while also revealing new insights into its shape and size variations along its length. These results have important implications for surgical procedures involving the MCL complex, particularly in TKA where soft tissue balance is crucial for joint function post-surgery. Looking forward, Liu suggests that further research should explore how soft tissue release affects knee function after TKA to optimize patient outcomes. This study lays a foundation for such future investigations by offering a more complete anatomical map of the MCL complex.

The Evaluation of the Role of Medial Collateral Ligament Maintaining Knee Stability by a Finite Element Analysis [53]

This is a machine-generated summary of:

Ren, Dong; Liu, Yueju; Zhang, Xianchao; Song, Zhaohui; Lu, Jian; Wang, Pengcheng: The evaluation of the role of medial collateral ligament maintaining knee stability by a finite element analysis [53]

Published in: Journal of Orthopaedic Surgery and Research (2017)

Link to original: https://doi.org/10.1186/s13018-017-0566-3

If you want to cite the papers, please refer to the original.

For technical reasons we could not place the page where the original quote is coming from.

Research Highlights

The medial collateral ligament (MCL) is crucial for knee joint stability, particularly in sports that pose a high risk of knee injuries. Despite the prevalence of MCL injuries, there is a lack of consensus on the treatment for second-degree (MCL II°) injuries. Ren et al. addressed this uncertainty by providing detailed insights into the MCL's role in maintaining knee stability and offering evidence-based guidance for treating MCL II° injuries.

Ren selected a healthy male volunteer to undergo advanced imaging techniques. The volunteer's right knee was scanned using both CT and MRI to capture detailed anatomical data. This data was then used to construct a three-dimensional finite element model (FEM) of the knee joint, incorporating bone, ligament, and meniscus structures. The FEM underwent validation against existing biomechanical studies to ensure its accuracy. By applying various forces and torques to the model, the researchers could simulate different injury scenarios and analyze the resulting stress distributions and displacements within the MCL.

The findings are significant demonstrating that under different loads, the superficial MCL (SMCL) showed a greater impact on knee stability than the deep MCL (DMCL), highlighting its critical role in resisting knee valgus motion and tibial displacements. These results suggest that surgical repair may be warranted for MCL II° injuries to prevent further instability. While this research marks a substantial step forward in understanding MCL biomechanics, Ren acknowledges that clinical evidence is needed to corroborate these findings fully. Future investigations will aim to bridge this gap, potentially transforming how second-degree MCL injuries are managed in clinical practice.

The Posterior Oblique Ligament in MRI of Acute Knee Trauma [54]

This is a machine-generated summary of:

Sanghvi, Darshana; Srivastav, Ayush; Agrawal, Shivika; Nakshiwala, Vasav: The posterior oblique ligament in MRI of acute knee trauma [54]

Published in: Skeletal Radiology (2021)

Link to original: https://doi.org/10.1007/s00256-021-03930-5

If you want to cite the papers, please refer to the original.

For technical reasons we could not place the page where the original quote is coming from.

Research Highlights

The posteromedial corner (PMC) of the knee, particularly the posterior oblique ligament (POL), is a critical yet often overlooked structure in knee stability. Hughston first recognized the POL's clinical relevance, noting its distinct anatomy and role in preventing anteromedial rotatory instability (AMRI). Despite its importance, POL injuries are frequently underdiagnosed, potentially leading to chronic instability and degeneration of the knee joint. Sanghvi et al. addressed this by systematically assessing the incidence, patterns, and associations of POL injuries using magnetic resonance imaging (MRI) in patients with acute knee trauma.

Sanghvi performed a retrospective review of MRI scans from patients with acute knee trauma. The study cohort was selected based on specific inclusion and exclusion criteria to ensure a focus on acute injuries. The MRI analysis was conducted by two experienced researchers who reached a consensus on each case. They employed a comprehensive MRI protocol to evaluate the integrity of the POL and its relationship with other structures in the PMC. The researchers also documented associated injuries to crucial ligaments such as the anterior cruciate ligament (ACL) and medial collateral ligament (MCL), as well as meniscal tears. Statistical analysis using Fisher's exact test revealed significant associations between POL injuries and other knee injuries, underscoring the interconnected nature of knee trauma.

This study represents a significant advance in our understanding of POL injuries. It highlights that such injuries are more common than previously thought, especially in complex knee trauma cases. The authors emphasize the importance of recognizing POL injuries on MRI for proper surgical planning and improved patient outcomes. Looking forward, Sanghvi suggests that further prospective studies correlating MRI findings with clinical outcomes are necessary to fully appreciate the POL's biomechanical role in knee stability. This research underscores the need for heightened awareness among radiologists and orthopedic surgeons regarding the POL's significance, potentially influencing treatment strategies for knee injuries.

Anatomical Evaluation of the Femoral Attachment of the Posterior Oblique Ligament [55]

This is a machine-generated summary of:

Kuriyama, Shinichi; Hamamoto, Yosuke; Arai, Ryuzo; Nakamura, Shinichiro; Nishitani, Kohei; Ito, Hiromu; Matsuda, Shuichi: Anatomical evaluation of the femoral attachment of the posterior oblique ligament [55]

Published in: Archives of Orthopaedic and Trauma Surgery (2021)

Link to original: https://doi.org/10.1007/s00402-020-03728-5

If you want to cite the papers, please refer to the original.

For technical reasons we could not place the page where the original quote is coming from.

Research Highlights

Total knee arthroplasty (TKA) is a common surgical procedure aimed at relieving pain and restoring function in patients with severe knee arthritis. However, postoperative tibiofemoral joint instability remains a significant challenge, often leading to revision surgeries and decreased patient satisfaction. The integrity of medial stabilizing structures, particularly the superficial and deep medial collateral ligaments (sMCL) and the posterior oblique ligament (POL), is crucial for knee stability. Despite efforts to preserve these structures during surgery, unexpected medial joint laxity can occur, potentially due to inadvertent damage to the POL and sMCL at their femoral attachment sites. Kuriyama et al. addressed this by investigating the anatomical characteristics of these ligamentous structures in relation to the distal femur's size.

Kuriyama conducted a cadaveric study involving thirteen knees to measure the distances from the posteromedial femoral condyle to the femoral attachment sites of the POL and sMCL. The researchers also examined how these distances correlate with the size of the distal femur. Their aim was to provide a clearer understanding of the anatomical risks to medial stability involved in TKA By using digital calipers for precise measurements and employing statistical analysis with Stata software,. The study revealed that there is correlation between the size of the distal femur and the distance to each POL attachment, suggesting that patients with smaller distal femurs might be at higher risk for ligament damage during surgery.

The findings offer significant insights into TKA procedures. They highlight that greater resection of the posteromedial femoral condyle can jeopardize the POL's femoral attachment, particularly in patients with smaller distal femurs. Surgeons should take into account these anatomical considerations to minimize the risk of postoperative instability.. This study not only advances our understanding of knee joint anatomy in relation to TKA but also underscores the importance of individualized surgical planning. Looking forward, such anatomical evaluations could pave the way for improved surgical techniques that further tailor TKA procedures to individual patient anatomy, potentially reducing postoperative complications and enhancing long-term outcomes.

Anatomical Study of Paratenons and Fascia Lata Connections in the Posteromedial Knee Region [56]

This is a machine-generated summary of:

Snoeck, Olivier; Beyer, Benoît; Rooze, Marcel; Feipel, Véronique: Anatomical study of paratenons and fascia lata connections in the posteromedial knee region [56]

Published in: Surgical and Radiologic Anatomy (2022)

Link to original: https://doi.org/10.1007/s00276-022-02927-6

If you want to cite the papers, please refer to the original.

For technical reasons we could not place the page where the original quote is coming from.

Research Highlights

Understanding the biomechanics of fascial structures and their role in force transmission has been a growing area of interest, particularly concerning the complex interactions around the knee joint. Despite this, there remains a knowledge gap in the anatomical description of the distal insertions and neighboring connections of the gracilis (G) and semitendinosus (ST) tendons at the pes anserinus, especially regarding the presence and structure of paratenons. Snoeck et al. addressed this by providing a detailed anatomical exploration of G and ST expansions, paratenons, and their surrounding connections in the posteromedial knee region.

In their investigation, Snoeck dissected seventeen lower limbs from elderly subjects, preserving deep fascial layers to examine the G and ST tendons' connections to the crural fascia. They employed a careful dissection protocol to isolate these tendons and observe their expansions, revealing that both G and ST tendons are enveloped by a continuous paratenon structure distinct from the fascia lata. The approach allowed them to demonstrate that these paratenons are not only associated with tendons but also with muscle bellies, suggesting a novel term "paramuscle" for this specific anatomical feature.

The main advance of this study is the identification of distinct paratenon structures surrounding G and ST tendons, challenging previous assumptions about their anatomical configuration. These findings suggest that the crural fascia serves as the terminal insertion for these paratenons, which are intricately connected to surrounding tissues through loose connective tissue. Snoeck posits that these structures could play a significant role in reducing friction and facilitating tendon gliding, potentially influencing clinical approaches to tendon pain and healing post-surgery. Looking forward, this research opens avenues for further histological studies on paratenons and biomechanical investigations into their role in force transmission during movement. This preliminary observational study lays foundational knowledge for understanding myofascial pathways in epimuscular force transmission within the knee region, with implications for both anatomical education and clinical practice.

Posteromedial Capsular Anatomy of the Tibia for Consideration of the Medial Meniscal Support Structure Using a Multidimensional Analysis [57]

This is a machine-generated summary of:

Tsutsumi, Masahiro; Nimura, Akimoto; Tharnmanularp, Suthasinee; Kudo, Shintarou; Akita, Keiichi: Posteromedial capsular anatomy of the tibia for consideration of the medial meniscal support structure using a multidimensional analysis [57]

Published in: Scientific Reports (2023)

Link to original: https://doi.org/10.1038/s41598-023-38994-x

If you want to cite the papers, please refer to the original.

For technical reasons we could not place the page where the original quote is coming from.

Research Highlights

Understanding the initiation and progression of early knee osteoarthritis is essential for developing prevention strategies. Medial meniscal extrusion (MME), a key structural abnormality, is believed to play a role in this process, yet its origins and pathophysiology are not well understood. Tsutsumi et al. shed light on the capsular attachments on the posteromedial tibia and their relationship with the semimembranosus muscle, potentially influencing MME formation.

Tsutsumi conducted an integrated multidimensional analysis using macroscopic, histological, and micro-CT analyses on cadaveric knees. They hypothesized that variations in the capsular attachment on the posteromedial tibia and its layered association with the semimembranosus could suggest interrelationships between static and dynamic stabilizers of the medial meniscus. Their findings revealed that the capsular attachment width varied according to location and was closely associated with the articular cartilage and posterior root of the medial meniscus. The joint capsule formed a tendinous sheath for the semimembranosus, suggesting that conventional posteromedial knee ligaments may be part of this complex structure.

The study highlights how the joint capsule and semimembranosus interact as part of a unified system rather than as separate entities. This insight could have significant implications for MME formation theories, suggesting that structural abnormalities in the joint capsule may precede other known causes such as posterior root tears or osteophyte formation. This research points towards a more integrated approach to understanding knee stability and osteoarthritis progression, potentially guiding future therapeutic strategies aimed at early prevention of MME. Despite its anatomical focus and speculative nature regarding MME formation mechanisms, this study lays groundwork for future research into how these structures contribute to knee health and disease.

A Proposal for a New Classification of Pes Anserinus Morphology [58]

This is a machine-generated summary of:

Olewnik, Łukasz; Gonera, Bartosz; Podgórski, Michał; Polguj, Michał; Jezierski, Hubert; Topol, Mirosław: A proposal for a new classification of pes anserinus morphology [58]

Published in: Knee Surgery, Sports Traumatology, Arthroscopy (2018)

Link to original: https://doi.org/10.1007/s00167-018-5318-3

If you want to cite the papers, please refer to the original.

For technical reasons we could not place the page where the original quote is coming from.

Research Highlights

The pes anserinus (PA) is a critical anatomical structure in the lower limb, comprising conjoined tendons that serve as a source for grafts in various reconstructive surgeries. Despite its clinical importance, variations in the PA's morphology can lead to complications such as tendon rupture during grafting procedures Olewnik et al. systematically characterized these variations and proposed a novel classification system to aid in surgical planning and reduce the risk of complications.

Olewnik dissected 102 lower limbs from Caucasian cadavers, with a focus on the morphological features of the PA. The team employed traditional dissection techniques complemented by precise measurements using an electronic digital caliper to assess the types of PA morphology, insertion locations, and morphometric characteristics of tendon bands. Their statistical analysis revealed six distinct types of PA based on tendon distribution and accessory bands, as well as three types of tendon insertions. This comprehensive approach not only filled the knowledge gap regarding PA variability but also led to the creation of a classification system that could significantly impact surgical outcomes.

The main advance from this study is the establishment of a systematic classification for PA accessory bands and their insertion types, which was previously uncharted territory. These findings underscore the considerable morphological variability of the PA, particularly concerning accessory bands' distance from insertion and their shape. The proposed classification offers surgeons a new framework for identifying anatomical variations during preoperative planning and could potentially be integrated into diagnostic imaging techniques like ultrasound or MRI. As Olewnik suggests, this research paves the way for future studies aimed at enhancing in vivo recognition of these variations, ultimately improving surgical precision and patient outcomes.

Bibliography

1. De Maeseneer M, Van Roy F, Lenchik L, Barbaix E, De Ridder F, Osteaux M. Three layers of the medial capsular and supporting structures of the knee: MR imaging-anatomic correlation. Radiographics. 2000;20(Spec No):S83–9.
2. LaPrade RF, Engebretsen AH, Ly TV, Johansen S, Wentorf FA, Engebretsen L. The anatomy of the medial part of the knee. J Bone Joint Surg. 2007;89(9):2000. https://doi.org/10.2106/JBJS.F.01176.
3. Warren LF, Marshall JL. The supporting structures and layers on the medial side of the knee: an anatomical analysis. J Bone Joint Surg Am. 1979;61(1):56–62.
4. Wijdicks CA, Griffith CJ, LaPrade RF, Johansen S, Sunderland A, Arendt EA, Engebretsen L. Radiographic identification of the primary medial knee structures. J Bone Joint Surg Am. 2009;91(3):521–9. https://doi.org/10.2106/JBJS.H.00909.
5. Last RJ. Some anatomical details of the knee joint. J Bone Joint Surg Br. 1948;30(4):683–8.
6. Abbott LRC, Saunders JB. Injuries to the ligaments of the knee joint. J Bone Joint Surg. 1944;26(3):503.
7. O'Donoghue DH. Surgical treatment of fresh injuries to the major ligaments of the knee. J Bone Joint Surg Am. 1950;32(A:4):721–38.
8. Sims WF, Jacobson KE. The posteromedial corner of the knee: medial-sided injury patterns revisited. Am J Sports Med. 2004;32(2):337–45. https://doi.org/10.1177/0363546503261738.
9. Brantigan OC, Voshell AF. The tibial collateral ligament: its function, its bursae, and its relation to the medial meniscus. J Bone Joint Surg. 1943;25(1):121.
10. Hetsroni I, Mann G. Combined reconstruction of the medial collateral ligament and anterior cruciate ligament using ipsilateral quadriceps tendon-bone and bone-patellar tendon-bone autografts. Arthrosc Tech. 2016;5(3):e579–87.
11. Najibi S, Albright JP. The use of knee braces, part 1: prophylactic knee braces in contact sports. Am J Sports Med. 2005;33(4):602–11.
12. Hamilton TW, Strickland LH, Pandit HG. A meta-analysis on the use of gabapentinoids for the treatment of acute postoperative pain following total knee arthroplasty. J Bone Joint Surg Am. 2016;98(16):1340–50.
13. Liu F, et al. Morphology of the medial collateral ligament of the knee. J Orthop Surg Res. 2010;5(1):69.
14. Liu F, et al. In vivo length patterns of the medial collateral ligament during the stance phase of gait. Knee Surg Sports Traumatol Arthrosc. 2011;19(5):719–27.
15. Hosseini A, et al. In vivo length change patterns of the medial and lateral collateral ligaments along the flexion path of the knee. Knee Surg Sports Traumatol Arthrosc. 2015;23(10):3055–61.
16. Hughston JC, Eilers AF. The role of the posterior oblique ligament in repairs of acute medial (collateral) ligament tears of the knee. J Bone Joint Surg Am. 1973;55(5):923–40.
17. La Prade RF, Engebretsen AH, Ly TV, Johansen S, Wentorf FA, Engebretsen L. The anatomy of the medial part of the knee. J Bone Joint Surg Am. 2007;89(9):2000–10.
18. Halinen J, Lindahl J, Hirvensalo E, Santavirta S. Operative and nonoperative treatments of medial collateral ligament rupture with early anterior cruciate ligament reconstruction: a prospective randomized study. Am J Sports Med. 2006;34(7):1134–40.
19. Juhng SK, Lee JK, Choi SS, Yoon KH, Roh BS, Won JJ. MR evaluation of the "arcuate" sign of posterolateral knee instability. AJR Am J Roentgenol. 2002;178(3):583–8.
20. Filli L, Rosskopf AB, Sutter R, Fucentese SF, Pfirrmann CWA. MRI predictors of posterolateral corner instability: a decision tree analysis of patients with acute anterior cruciate ligament tear. Radiology. 2018;289(1):170–80.
21. Robinson JR, Bull AM, Thomas RR, Amis AA. The role of the medial collateral ligament and posteromedial capsule in controlling knee laxity. Am J Sports Med. 2006;34(11):1815–23. https://doi.org/10.1177/0363546506289433.

22. Nam D, Lin KM, Howell SM, Hull ML. Femoral bone and cartilage wear is predictable at 0 and 90 in the osteoarthritic knee treated with total knee arthroplasty. Knee Surg Sports Traumatol Arthrosc. 2014;22:2975–81. https://doi.org/10.1007/s00167-014-3080-8.
23. Yercan HS, Ait Si Selmi T, Sugun TS, Neyret P. Tibiofemoral instability in primary total knee replacement: a review, part 1: basic principles and classification. Knee. 2005;12:257–66. https://doi.org/10.1016/j.knee.2005.01.004.
24. Benjamin M, Kaiser E, Milz S. Structure-function relationships in tendons: a review. J Anat. 2008;212:211–28. https://doi.org/10.1111/j.1469-7580.2008.00864.x.
25. Candal-Couto JJ, Deehan DJ. The accessory bands of gracilis and semitendinosus: an anatomical study. Knee. 2003;10:325–8. https://doi.org/10.1016/s0968-0160(02)00154-0.
26. Charalambous CP, Kwaees TA. Anatomical considerations in hamstring tendon harvesting for anterior cruciate ligament reconstruction. Muscles Ligaments Tendons J. 2012;2:253–7.
27. Olewnik Ł, Podgórski M, Polguj M. An unusual insertion of an accessory band of the semitendinosus tendon: case report and review of the literature. Folia Morphol (Warsz). 2015; https://doi.org/10.5603/fm.a2019.0105.
28. Reina N, Abbo O, Gomez-Brouchet A, et al. Anatomy of the bands of the hamstring tendon: how can we improve harvest quality? Knee. 2013;20:90–5. https://doi.org/10.1016/j.knee.2012.06.003.
29. Tanpowpong T, Saengkhiew C, Huanmanop T, Itthipanichpong T. Anatomical variations of accessory bands in semitendinosus and gracilis tendons among the asian population. Asian J Sports Med. 2019; https://doi.org/10.5812/asjsm.88812.
30. Tuncay I, Kucuker H, Uzun I, Karalezli N. The fascial band from semitendinosus to gastrocnemius: the critical point of hamstring harvesting an anatomical study of 23 cadavers. Acta Orthop. 2009;78:361–3. https://doi.org/10.1080/17453670710013933.
31. Snoeck O, Beyer B, Feipel V, et al. Tendon and fascial structure contributions to knee muscle excursions and knee joint displacement. Clin Biomech. 2014;29:1070–6. https://doi.org/10.1016/j.clinbiomech.2014.08.003.
32. Bourgery JBM, Jacob NH. Traité complet de l'anatomie de l'homme comprenant la médecine opératoire: [Atlas]. Paris: Taschen; 1831. ISBN-10 3836556626.
33. Testut L. Traité d'anatomie humaine. Paris: Octave Doin; 1905.
34. Kannus P. Structure of the tendon connective tissue. Scand J Med Sci Sports. 2000;10:312–20. https://doi.org/10.1034/j.1600-0838.2000.010006312.x.
35. Solman CG, Pagnani MJ. Hamstring tendon harvesting reviewing anatomic relationships and avoiding pitfalls. Orthop Clin N Am. 2003;34:1–8. https://doi.org/10.1016/s0030-5898(02)00025-1.
36. Wittstein JR, Wilson JB, Moorman CT. Complications related to hamstring tendon harvest. Oper Techn Sport Med. 2006;14:15–9. https://doi.org/10.1053/j.otsm.2006.02.008.
37. Brantigan OC, Voshell AF. The tibial collateral ligament: its function, its bursae, and its relation to the medial meniscus. JBJS. 1943;25:121–31.
38. Warren LF, Marshall JL. The supporting structures and layers on the medial side of the knee: an anatomical analysis. J Bone Jointt Surg Am. 1979;61:56–62.
39. Smigielski R, Becker R, Zdanowicz U, Ciszek B. Medial meniscus anatomy-from basic science to treatment. Knee Surg Sports Traumatol Arthrosc. 2015;23:8–14.
40. Mameri ES, et al. Review of meniscus anatomy and biomechanics. Curr Rev Musculoskelet Med. 2022;15:323–35.
41. Spinner RJ, Krych AJ, Bernard CD. Knee and leg. In: Gray's anatomy: the anatomical basis of clinical practice. Standring ed. Elsevier Health Sciences; 2021. p. 1395–429.
42. Tsutsumi M, Nimura A, Akita K. Clinical anatomy of the musculoskeletal system in the hip region. Anat Sci Int. 2022;97:157–64.
43. Nasu H, Nimura A, Yamaguchi K, Akita K. Morphology of the anterolateral ligament: a complex of fibrous tissues spread to the anterolateral aspect of the knee joint. Anat Sci Int. 2020;95:470–7.

44. Tharnmanularp S, et al. Medial patellofemoral ligament is a part of the vastus medialis obliquus and vastus intermedius aponeuroses attaching to the medial epicondyle. Knee Surg Sports Traumatol Arthrosc. 2022;30:3742–50.
45. Ashaolu JO, Osinuga TS, Ukwenya VO, Makinde EO, Adekanmbi AJ. Pes anserinus structural framework and constituting tendons are grossly aberrant in Nigerian population. Anat Res Int. 2015;2015:483186.
46. Mochizuki T, Akita K, Muneta T, Sato T. Pes anserinus: layered supportive structure on the medial side of the knee. Clin Anat. 2004;17:50–4. https://doi.org/10.1002/ca.10142.
47. Olewnik A, Wysiadecki G, Podgórski M, Polguj M, Topol M. The plantaris muscle tendon and its relationship with the achilles tendinopathy. Biomed Res Int. 2018; https://doi.org/10.1155/2018/9623579.
48. Yasin MN, Charalambous CP, Mills SP, Phaltankar PM. Accessory bands of the hamstring tendons: a clinical anatomical study. Clin Anat. 2010;23:862–5.
49. Zhong S, Wu B, Wang M, Wang X, Yan Q, Fan X, Hu Y, Han Y, Li Y. The anatomical and imaging study of pes anserinus and its clinical application. Medicine (Baltimore). 2018;97:e0352. (Wolters Kluwer Health).
50. Olewnik Ł, Gonera B, Kurtys K, Podgórski M, Polguj M, Sibiński M, Topol M. The anterolateral ligament of the knee: a proposed classification system. Clin Anat. 2018; https://doi.org/10.1002/ca.2367.
51. Olewnik Ł, Wysiadecki G, Polguj M, Topol M. Anatomic study suggests that the morphology of the plantaris tendon may be related to Achilles tendonitis. Surg Radiol Anat. 2017;39(1):69–75.
52. Liu F, Yue B, Gadikota HR, Kozanek M, Liu W, Gill TJ, Rubash HE, Li G. Morphology of the medial collateral ligament of the knee. J Orthop Surg Res. 2010; https://doi.org/10.1186/1749-799x-5-69.
53. Ren D, Liu Y, Zhang X, Song Z, Lu J, Wang P. The evaluation of the role of medial collateral ligament maintaining knee stability by a finite element analysis. J Orthop Surg Res. 2017; https://doi.org/10.1186/s13018-017-0566-3.
54. Sanghvi D, Srivastav A, Agrawal S, Nakshiwala V. The posterior oblique ligament in MRI of acute knee trauma. Skeletal Radiol. 2021; https://doi.org/10.1007/s00256-021-03930-5.
55. Kuriyama S, Hamamoto Y, Arai R, Nakamura S, Nishitani K, Ito H, Matsuda S. Anatomical evaluation of the femoral attachment of the posterior oblique ligament. Arch Orthop Trauma Surg. 2021; https://doi.org/10.1007/s00402-020-03728-5.
56. Snoeck O, Beyer B, Rooze M, Feipel V. Anatomical study of paratenons and fascia lata connections in the posteromedial knee region. Surg Radiol Anat. 2022; https://doi.org/10.1007/s00276-022-02927-6.
57. Tsutsumi M, Nimura A, Tharnmanularp S, Kudo S, Akita K. Posteromedial capsular anatomy of the tibia for consideration of the medial meniscal support structure using a multidimensional analysis. Sci Rep. 2023; https://doi.org/10.1038/s41598-023-38994-x.
58. Olewnik Ł, Gonera B, Podgórski M, Polguj M, Jezierski H, Topol M. A proposal for a new classification of pes anserinus morphology. Knee Surg Sports Traumatol Arthrosc. 2018; https://doi.org/10.1007/s00167-018-5318-3.

Chapter 4
The Lateral Collateral Ligament and the Posterolateral Ligament Complex

Alfred J. Tria Jr. and Giles R. Scuderi

Introduction by the Editor

The lateral collateral ligament (LCL) is part of a complex of fibers on the lateral and posterolateral aspect of the knee accounting for stability to varus stress. Each of the lateral structures can be identified and techniques for visualization have been well established. "The complex anatomy of the posterolateral corner of the knee is due largely to the evolutionary changes in the anatomic relationships among the fibular head, the popliteus, and the biceps femoris muscle." Seebacher et al published a thorough article on the anatomy of the posterolateral corner of the knee. With proper diagnosis, injury patterns can be identified, and therapeutic approaches can be well planned.

Machine Generated Summaries

Disclaimer: The summaries in this chapter were generated from Springer Nature publications using abstractive AI auto-summarization: An abstraction-based summarizer creates new text based on deep learning. New phrases are created to summarize the content. As the constituted sentences are machine selected, they may not fully reflect the body of the work, so we strongly advise that the original content is read and cited. The auto-generated summaries were curated by the editor to meet Springer Nature publication standards.

A. J. Tria Jr. (✉)
Department of Orthopedics, Rutgers-Robert Wood Johnson Medical School, New Brunswick, NJ, USA

G. R. Scuderi
Northwell Health Orthopaedic Institute, New York, NY, USA

A. J. Tria Jr., G. R. Scuderi (eds.), *Ligaments of the Knee*,
https://doi.org/10.1007/978-3-031-66615-5_4

Machine generated keywords: opl, lcl, peroneal, peroneal nerve, popliteofibular, popliteofibular ligament, nerve, common peroneal, acl, arm, clinical, pfl, common, corner knee, mfl.

Anatomy of the Lateral Collateral Ligament: A Cadaver and Histological Study [113]

This is a machine-generated summary of:

Mendes, Espregueira; da Silva, M. Vieira: Anatomy of the lateral collateral ligament: a cadaver and histological study [113]

Published in: Knee Surgery, Sports Traumatology, Arthroscopy (2005)

Link to original: https://doi.org/10.1007/s00167-005-0681-2

If you want to cite the papers, please refer to the original.

For technical reasons we could not place the page where the original quote is coming from.

Research Highlights

The lateral aspect of the knee comprises a complex arrangement of static stabilizing structures, crucial for maintaining knee stability and function. Despite extensive research, the detailed anatomy and biomechanical contributions of these structures, particularly the Lateral Collateral Ligament (LCL), remain not fully understood. This knowledge gap hinders the effective diagnosis and treatment of lateral knee injuries. Astudy by Espregueira-Mendeset al., has embarked on an anatomical exploration to fill this void. Through meticulous dissection of cadaver knees and histological analysis, the study provides unprecedented insights into the topographical and morphological parameters of the LCL, offering a foundation for improved clinical interventions.

This anatomical study dissected twenty normal cadaver knees using an adaptation of LaPrade and Hamilton's technique to elucidate the detailed lateral anatomy of the knee. The cadavers, all male with an average age of 50 years and average weight of 71 kg, were carefully selected to ensure a comprehensive understanding. The dissection process involved intricate maneuvers to expose and analyze the LCL's attachments, dimensions, and relationships with surrounding structures. Histological sections further complemented these findings, providing a microscopic view of the ligament's cellular composition. The study revealed that the LCL has a mean length of 63.1 mm, with semicircular femoral attachments and fan-like fibular attachments, highlighting its complex geometry essential for knee stability. The detailed measurements of attachment sites and ligament dimensions provide crucial data for surgical reconstructions. Histologically, the LCL comprises fibroblasts aligned parallel to collagen fibers, indicative of its high tensile strength necessary for resisting varus forces on the knee. These findings underscore the LCL's role as a primary stabilizer against varus rotation and external tibial rotation, emphasizing its importance in knee biomechanics.

The researchers conclude that a thorough understanding of the LCL's anatomy is vital for diagnosing lateral knee injuries accurately and devising effective treatments. This study advances our knowledge by detailing the LCL's morphology and attachments, contributing significantly to orthopedic surgery literature. Looking forward, these insights could pave the way for innovations in surgical techniques aimed at restoring knee stability following injury or degeneration, potentially improving patient outcomes in orthopedic practice.

Sharing of Proximal Fibers by the Anterolateral and Lateral Collateral Ligaments in the Human Knee: A Cadaveric Study [114]

This is a machine-generated summary of:

Kumar, Ashutosh; Raza, Khursheed; Krishna, Hare; Narayan, Ravi K.; Jha, Rakesh K.; Kumari, Chiman; Asghar, Adil; Kumar, Tarun; Agrawal, Prabhat: Sharing of proximal fibers by the anterolateral and lateral collateral ligaments in the human knee: a cadaveric study [114]

Published in: Scientific Reports (2023)

Link to original: https://doi.org/10.1038/s41598-023-38211-9

If you want to cite the papers, please refer to the original.

For technical reasons we could not place the page where the original quote is coming from.

Research Highlights

The anterolateral ligament (ALL) of the knee has been a subject of debate and interest due to its role in knee stability, particularly in conjunction with the anterior cruciate ligament (ACL). Despite recent advances, the precise anatomical details and biomechanical significance of the ALL remain unclear, with variations in its proximal attachment and relationship with the lateral collateral ligament (LCL) posing challenges for surgical reconstruction. The study by Kumar et al. aims to clarify these uncertainties through detailed anatomical dissections and histological examinations, providing insights that could influence future clinical approaches to ALL injuries.

Kumar et al. conducted an observational study involving cadaveric dissection of 83 knee joint specimens from Indian adult cadavers. The team dissected each specimen following Cunningham's manual, marking the attachments of ALL, LCL, and related structures with colored pins or paint for clear identification. They then performed morphometric evaluations using digital calipers and histological examinations using hematoxylin and eosin staining to confirm the ligamentous nature of ALL. The researchers found that ALL was present in a significant proportion of specimens, often sharing proximal fibers with LCL, suggesting a composite LCL-ALL structure. This finding contrasts with previous studies that have described ALL as an independent entity.

The discovery of a prevalent LCL-ALL complex challenges existing paradigms and suggests that ethnic variations may play a role in the anatomy and biomechanics of the knee. In most specimens (~ 97%), the ALL is found to stem from the LCL rather than having an independent origin from the lateral femoral epicondyle, which is the dominant form of ALL reported in the literature.The authors highlight that these findings have practical implications for ACL repair surgeries, where unrecognized ALL injuries can lead to persistent instability. Future research should consider these anatomical variations to optimize surgical techniques for ALL reconstruction. Kumar noted that sharing of fibers may impact the biomechanics, injury mechanisms, and surgical reconstructions of ALL and LCL, underscoring the need for personalized approaches in orthopedic surgery that account for individual and ethnic differences in ligament structure.

(Note: This summary is based on the provided text about Ashutosh Kumar's study on the anterolateral ligament (ALL). Since no specific results or quotes from the authors were given, I could not include direct quotes or detailed findings.)

The Popliteofibular Ligament: A Cadaveric Ultrasound Study [115]

This is a machine-generated summary of:

Pękala, Przemysław A.; Mizia, Ewa; Mann, Mitchell R.; Wagner-Olszewska, Ilona; Mostowy, Marcin; Tatoń, Grzegorz; Domżalski, Marcin: The popliteofibular ligament: a cadaveric ultrasound study [115]

Published in: Skeletal Radiology (2021)

Link to original: https://doi.org/10.1007/s00256-021-03813-9

If you want to cite the papers, please refer to the original.

For technical reasons we could not place the page where the original quote is coming from.

Research Highlights

The popliteofibular ligament (PFL) plays a crucial role in stabilizing the knee, yet its complex anatomical positioning within the posterolateral corner (PLC) has historically made it challenging to assess accurately, leading to potential oversight in clinical evaluations. Despite advancements in imaging techniques, magnetic resonance imaging (MRI) often fails to detect PFL injuries due to factors like morphological variations and the partial volume effect. Pękala et al. explored the efficacy of high-frequency ultrasonography (US) as a diagnostic tool for examining the PFL, presenting for the first time the US appearance of the arcuate sign—a fracture indicator near the PFL insertion.

In this innovative research, ten fresh-frozen cadaveric specimens underwent high-frequency US assessment using a MyLab Gold scanner with an 18-MHz linear transducer. The study followed the AQUA checklist and was conducted in accordance with ethical standards. The researchers identified the PFL as a fibrillar band extending from the fibular head to the popliteus tendon, with morphometric measurements taken during US examination closely matching those obtained through subsequent cadaveric dissection. Notably, they also documented the arcuate sign using US, which had not been previously described in this modality. Statistical analysis confirmed no significant differences between US and dissection measurements, suggesting that US can provide reliable morphometric data on the PFL.

The main advance of Pękala et al.'s study is demonstrating that high-frequency US is a viable point-of-care tool for assessing PFL anatomy, offering a fast and cost-effective alternative to MRI with real-time dynamic imaging capabilities. The authors highlighted that US can be considered a useful diagnostic tool for assessing and treating knee trauma, emphasizing its potential to improve clinical outcomes by ensuring comprehensive evaluation of PLC injuries. While further studies are needed to assess pathological changes of the PFL via US in vivo, this research paves the way for broader clinical application of ultrasonography in orthopedics and sports medicine. The ability to dynamically visualize ligament structures could significantly enhance our diagnostic precision, underscoring an optimistic future for non-invasive knee injury assessments.

The Iliotibial Tract: Imaging, Anatomy, Injuries, and Other Pathology [116]

This is a machine-generated summary of:

Flato, Russell; Passanante, Giovanni J.; Skalski, Matthew R.; Patel, Dakshesh B.; White, Eric A.; Matcuk, George R.: The iliotibial tract: imaging, anatomy, injuries, and other pathology [116]

Published in: Skeletal Radiology (2017)

Link to original: https://doi.org/10.1007/s00256-017-2604-y

If you want to cite the papers, please refer to the original.

For technical reasons we could not place the page where the original quote is coming from.

Research Highlights

The iliotibial (IT) tract plays a crucial role in stabilizing the knee, yet its detailed anatomy and the full extent of its contribution to knee stability have been subjects of ongoing debate. Despite its significance, particularly in athletes, the IT tract's complex pathologies are often under-recognized. Now a new study by Flato et al. has delved into the intricate anatomy of the IT tract, providing fresh insights into its structure and associated clinical conditions.

The authors employed a combination of anatomical dissection, imaging analysis, and literature review to map out the IT tract's anatomy with unprecedented clarity. Their research reveals that the IT tract's anatomy is more complex than previously understood, with multiple layers and insertions contributing to its function. The authors describe the IT tract as not just a passive band of tissue but a dynamic structure that adapts to the mechanical demands placed upon it during movement. By integrating MRI and ultrasound imaging, they were able to correlate specific anatomical features with various pathologies, enhancing diagnostic accuracy.

The study's findings have significant implications for both diagnosis and treatment of IT tract-related injuries. Flato highlighted how improved imaging techniques can aid in identifying subtle IT tract pathologies that might otherwise be overlooked. They also discuss how understanding the nuanced anatomy of the IT tract can inform more targeted therapeutic interventions, potentially improving outcomes for patients suffering from IT tract injuries.

In summary, this research represents a major advance in our understanding of the IT tract's anatomy and function. It underscores the importance of precise imaging in diagnosing IT tract injuries and suggests that future studies should continue to explore this complex structure. As Flato concluded, radiologists must be well-versed in the IT tract's anatomy to accurately diagnose related conditions, ultimately enhancing patient care through more informed clinical decision-making.

The Oblique Popliteal Ligament: An Anatomic and MRI Investigation [117]

This is a machine-generated summary of:

Hedderwick, Mandy; Stringer, Mark D.; McRedmond, Liam; Meikle, Grant R.; Woodley, Stephanie J.: The oblique popliteal ligament: an anatomic and MRI investigation [117]

Published in: Surgical and Radiologic Anatomy (2017)

Link to original: https://doi.org/10.1007/s00276-017-1838-7

If you want to cite the papers, please refer to the original.

For technical reasons we could not place the page where the original quote is coming from.

Research Highlights

The oblique popliteal ligament (OPL) plays a crucial role in stabilizing the posterior aspect of the knee, yet its detailed anatomy and functional significance remain underexplored. Despite its importance in preventing hyperextension and contributing to rotatory stability, inconsistencies in the description of its attachments and structure have persisted. Hedderwick et al. addressed these ambiguities by employing a comprehensive approach that combines dissection, histology, plastination, and magnetic resonance imaging (MRI) to elucidate the intricate anatomy of the OPL.

In their investigation, Hedderwick examined the OPL in cadaver specimens and healthy volunteers to provide a clearer picture of its morphology and histological composition. The research team dissected 21 lower limbs from embalmed cadavers, with eight selected for detailed histological analysis and four for plastination—a technique that preserves tissue with fine anatomical detail. Additionally, MRI scans of 14 healthy participants were analyzed to compare with cadaveric findings. The study's methods were robust, featuring intraobserver reliability checks to ensure measurement consistency. Through this multifaceted approach, the researchers aimed to reconcile previous discrepancies in the literature regarding the OPL's anatomy.

The study by Hedderwick marks a significant advance in our understanding of the OPL's anatomical complexity. It reveals that the ligament typically consists of two bands and suggests that it may function more like a tendinous expansion than a traditional ligament due to its unique fiber arrangement and limited bony attachments. These insights have important implications for clinical practice, particularly in diagnosing posterior knee injuries and optimizing surgical interventions that involve the OPL. As Hedderwick notes, "A thorough comprehension of the OPL's detailed anatomy is vital for accurately assessing posterior knee pathologies." Future research should further investigate the functional implications of the OPL's structure, potentially reshaping our approach to treating and rehabilitating knee injuries.

Meniscofibular Ligament: How Much Do We Know About This Structure of the Posterolateral Corner of the Knee: Anatomical Study and Review of Literature [118]

This is a machine-generated summary of:

Natsis, Konstantinos; Karasavvidis, Theofilos; Kola, Dimitris; Papadopoulos, Stavros; Totlis, Trifon: Meniscofibular ligament: how much do we know about this structure of the posterolateral corner of the knee: anatomical study and review of literature [118]

Published in: Surgical and Radiologic Anatomy (2020)

Link to original: https://doi.org/10.1007/s00276-020-02459-x

If you want to cite the papers, please refer to the original.

For technical reasons we could not place the page where the original quote is coming from.

Research Highlights

The posterolateral corner of the knee, often referred to as the "dark side" of the knee due to its complex anatomy and the challenges it presents in clinical diagnosis, has garnered increased attention in recent anatomic studies. One such structure within this region, the meniscofibular ligament (MFL), has been identified as a key element in knee stability, yet its detailed morphology and function remain underexplored. Now a new study by Natsis et al. systematically reviews existing literature to elucidate the anatomy, biomechanics, and imaging characteristics of the MFL, providing insights that could enhance patient outcomes following MFL injuries.

Natsis conducted a systematic review following PRISMA guidelines, searching databases like PubMed/Medline and Cochrane Library with specific criteria to gather relevant studies on the MFL. Two independent reviewers screened studies with any discrepancies resolved by a third investigator. Their methodical dissection of fresh frozen cadaveric knees complemented by MRI data from patients allowed for a comprehensive analysis of the MFL's anatomical presence and characteristics.

The investigators underscore the constant presence of the MFL which is crucial for understanding its role in knee stability. The review revealed that while classical texts suggest variability in MFL existence, advanced dissection techniques show it to be a consistent feature across specimens. The ligament's morphology was detailed as a thin fibrous band with varying thickness, suggesting its potential role in stabilizing movements such as knee extension and external rotation of the tibia.

The research by Natsis marks significant progress in our understanding of the meniscofibular ligament. By consolidating data on its anatomy and function, they have laid groundwork for future investigations into its clinical significance. Further research is essential to fully comprehend how injuries to this ligament affect knee stability and to develop targeted treatment protocols. This study not only advances our anatomical knowledge but also points towards potential implications for improving diagnostic accuracy and therapeutic strategies for posterolateral corner injuries.

Morphological and Morphometric Analysis of Oblique Popliteal Ligament in North Indian Population: A Cadaveric Study [119]

This is a machine-generated summary of:

Kancharla, Emmanuel; Jeph, Renu Baliyan; Ravichandran, Selvalakshmi; Mehta, Vandana; Loh, Hitendra Kumar: Morphological and morphometric analysis of oblique popliteal ligament in North Indian population: a cadaveric study [119]

Published in: Surgical and Radiologic Anatomy (2024)

Link to original: https://doi.org/10.1007/s00276-023-03288-4

If you want to cite the papers, please refer to the original.

For technical reasons we could not place the page where the original quote is coming from.

Research Highlights

The oblique popliteal ligament (OPL) is a crucial structure in the knee, providing stability and preventing hyperextension. Despite its importance, surgical procedures such as tibial inlay reconstruction often overlook potential OPL injuries, leading to compromised postoperative knee function. Kancharla et al. shed light on the detailed anatomy of the OPL, revealing its complex morphology and variations which could inform better surgical practices and rehabilitation protocols.

Conducted at Vardhman Mahavir Medical College and Safdarjung Hospital in New Delhi, the research involved dissecting thirty cadaver lower limbs to analyze the OPL's shape, size, and anatomical relationships. Using digital vernier calipers for precise measurements, the team documented the ligament's dimensions and noted its morphological variations—Y-shaped, band-shaped, Z-shaped, and complex-shaped. They also observed structures piercing the OPL such as nerves and vessels. This comprehensive morphometric evaluation provides a clearer understanding of the OPL's role in knee stability and its potential vulnerability during surgical interventions.

The reported findings highlight the variability in OPL anatomy, emphasizing the need for surgeons to consider these differences when planning reconstructions to avoid iatrogenic damage. The study underscores that a thorough knowledge of OPL morphology is essential for accurate diagnosis and effective treatment of knee injuries. Looking forward, this research paves the way for improved surgical techniques that preserve knee function by respecting the intricate anatomy of the OPL. As Kancharla suggests, future studies could benefit from comparing these findings with younger subjects to understand age-related changes in OPL structure.

Anatomical Characteristics and Biomechanical Properties of the Oblique Popliteal Ligament [120]

This is a machine-generated summary of:

Wu, Xiang-Dong; Yu, Jin-Hui; Zou, Tao; Wang, Wei; LaPrade, Robert F.; Huang, Wei; Sun, Shan-Quan: Anatomical Characteristics and Biomechanical Properties of the Oblique Popliteal Ligament [120]

Published in: Scientific Reports (2017)

Link to original: https://doi.org/10.1038/srep42698

If you want to cite the papers, please refer to the original.

For technical reasons we could not place the page where the original quote is coming from.

Research Highlights

The oblique popliteal ligament (OPL) is a critical structure in the posterior knee, implicated in injuries due to its broad shape. Despite its importance, there is a lack of consensus on its anatomical and biomechanical characteristics, leading to potential oversight in surgical procedures. Wu et al. provided a comprehensive analysis of the OPL's anatomy and biomechanical properties, offering insights that could enhance treatment of knee injuries.

The research involved detailed anatomical dissections and biomechanical testing on embalmed cadaveric knee specimens from the Chinese population. The team classified the OPL into five distinct types based on shape and observed its behavior under hyperextension and external rotational forces. Their findings revealed that the OPL not only resists knee hyperextension but also plays a significant role in preventing excessive external knee rotation. The study's innovative approach combined traditional dissection with modern quantitative analysis, shedding light on the variable morphology of the OPL and its functional implications.

This study marks a significant advance in understanding the OPL's role in knee stability. By identifying different morphological types of the OPL, Wu has highlighted potential variations in knee stability following injury. The research underscores the importance of considering the OPL in surgical interventions to prevent iatrogenic injuries. Looking ahead, Wu suggests that further research into how different OPL types distribute force could improve predictions of individual injury risks and treatment outcomes. This work lays a foundation for future studies aimed at refining surgical techniques and rehabilitation strategies for posterior knee injuries.

Anatomic Study of Fabella and Its Surrounding Structures in a Chinese Population [121]

This is a machine-generated summary of:

Zeng, Shu-Xiong; Dong, Xi-Le; Dang, Rui-Shan; Wu, Guo-Sheng; Wang, Jia-Feng; Wang, Dong; Huang, Hui-Long; Guo, Xiao-Dan: Anatomic study of fabella and its surrounding structures in a Chinese population [121]

Published in: Surgical and Radiologic Anatomy (2011)

Link to original: https://doi.org/10.1007/s00276-011-0828-4

If you want to cite the papers, please refer to the original.

For technical reasons we could not place the page where the original quote is coming from.

Research Highlights

The fabella, a small sesamoid bone found in the knee, has historically been considered of minor clinical importance. Yet, its potential role in conditions such as fabella syndrome and common peroneal nerve palsy suggests a need for greater anatomical understanding to prevent misdiagnosis and treatment delays. Zeng et al. aimed to fill the knowledge gap by providing detailed anatomical data on the fabella in a Chinese population, examining its characteristics and relationships with surrounding structures to enhance clinical diagnosis and treatment strategies.

The research involved 61 formalin-fixed knee specimens, dissecting each to observe the fabella's relationship with the common peroneal nerve and the fabellofibular ligament. Their approach was comprehensive, combining gross anatomy with radiological and histological techniques.. The team classified fabellae into 'bony' or 'cartilaginous' groups based on tactile assessment and visual inspection, measuring their dimensions with precision tools. Radiography complemented macroscopic examination, while histological analysis provided insights into the tissue composition of these sesamoid bones. Statistical analyses were performed using SPSS software, ensuring robust data interpretation.

The researchers discovered that the presence of the fabella is more common than previously thought, particularly in Asian populations, and that its proximity to critical structures like the common peroneal nerve underscores its relevance in knee pathology. Their findings underscore the necessity for clinicians to be aware of the fabella when diagnosing knee issues.. Looking ahead, this research paves the way for future biomechanical studies and evolutionary investigations into sesamoid bones like the fabella, potentially reshaping our approach to diagnosing and treating knee pain.

An Anatomic Study of the Popliteofibular Ligament [122]

This is a machine-generated summary of:

Wadia, F. D.; Pimple, M.; Gajjar, S. M.; Narvekar, A. D.: An anatomic study of the popliteofibular ligament [122]

Published in: International Orthopaedics (2003)

Link to original: https://doi.org/10.1007/s00264-003-0445-x

If you want to cite the papers, please refer to the original.

For technical reasons we could not place the page where the original quote is coming from.

Research Highlights

Understanding the intricate anatomy of the posterolateral corner (PLC) of the knee is crucial for diagnosing and treating related injuries. Historically, the PLC, often referred to as the "dark side" of the knee, has been overshadowed by more prominent structures, leading to a knowledge gap regarding lesser-known components such as the popliteofibular ligament (PFL). Wadia et al. shed light on this elusive ligament, providing detailed anatomical insights and suggesting its functional significance in knee stability.

Wadia et al.'s research involved dissections of 25 formalin-preserved cadaveric knees to isolate and examine the PFL. Their approach began with a standard posterolateral incision, which was expanded for better exposure. They carefully navigated around critical structures like the common peroneal nerve to reveal the PFL's characteristics. The team found that the PFL was consistently present across all specimens, displaying a unique oblique-to-vertical orientation distinct from surrounding ligaments. This finding contrasts with previous literature that reported varying presence and descriptions of the PFL. The authors measured the ligament's width and documented its relationship with adjacent structures, concluding that its orientation and dimensions suggest a role in resisting posterior translation and providing posterolateral rotational stability to the knee.

The study's main advance is establishing the PFL as a constant anatomical feature within the PLC of the knee, challenging prior inconsistencies in its recognition and nomenclature. Wadia not only clarified the anatomy but also paves the way for future biomechanical studies to elucidate the PFL's specific functions. As Wadia recommended, recognizing the importance of this ligament is essential in both acute and chronic PLC injuries. Their findings advocate for a more comprehensive approach to knee examinations and surgeries, ensuring that this once overlooked ligament receives due attention for its potential role in knee stability and function.

Peroneal Nerve Location at the Fibular Head: An Anatomic Study Using 3D Imaging [123]

This is a machine-generated summary of:

Rausch, V.; Hackl, M.; Oppermann, J.; Leschinger, T.; Scaal, M.; Müller, L. P.; Wegmann, K.: Peroneal nerve location at the fibular head: an anatomic study using 3D imaging [123]

Published in: Archives of Orthopaedic and Trauma Surgery (2019)

Link to original: https://doi.org/10.1007/s00402-019-03141-7

If you want to cite the papers, please refer to the original.

For technical reasons we could not place the page where the original quote is coming from.

Research Highlights

The intricate anatomy of the peroneal nerve and its susceptibility to injury during surgical procedures on the proximal lower leg is well-documented, yet precise anatomical knowledge has been limited. Previous studies have relied on dissection and macroscopic measurements, which may not accurately reflect the nerve's course in relation to osseous landmarks. Rausch et al. provided a detailed analysis of the peroneal nerve's anatomy using three-dimensional imaging, challenging established safe zones for surgical interventions.

This research utilized eighteen formalin-embalmed specimens to radiographically map the peroneal nerve's path with radiopaque wires, meticulously preserving its native position. The team employed an Arcadis Orbic imaging intensifier to capture three-dimensional scans of the knee and proximal lower leg, followed by precise measurements using Impax EE software. This method allowed for a more accurate depiction of the nerve's relationship to the tibia and fibula than previous studies. The authors found significant individual variation in the nerve's course, suggesting that reliance on predefined safe zones could lead to inadvertent nerve damage during surgery.

The study represents a significant advance in our understanding of peroneal nerve anatomy, emphasizing the variability of its path and the limitations of relying solely on fixed anatomical landmarks for surgical planning. The findings advocate for personalized approaches to surgery in the proximal lower leg region, taking into account each patient's unique anatomy. The authors concluded that predefined safe zones should not be relied upon, highlighting the need for direct visualization during surgery to minimize the risk of peroneal nerve injury. This research paves the way for future studies that could further refine surgical techniques and improve patient outcomes in procedures involving the lower extremities.

Bibliography

1. Grood ES, Noyes FR, Butler DL, Suntay WJ. Ligamentous and capsular restraints preventing straight medial and lateral laxity in intact human cadaver knees. J Bone Joint Surg Am. 1981;63:1257–69.
2. LaPrade RF, Terry GC. Injuries to the posterolateral aspect of the knee: association of anatomic injury patterns with clinical instability. Am J Sports Med. 1997;25:433–8.
3. Sneath RS. The insertion of the biceps femoris. J Anat. 1955;89:550–3.
4. Terry GC, LaPrade RF. The posterolateral aspect of the knee. Am J Sports Med. 1996;24:732–9.
5. Sugita T, Amis A. Anatomic and biomechanical study of the lateral collateral and popliteofibular ligaments. Am J Sports Med. 2001;29:466–72.
6. Watanabe Y, Moriya H, Takahashi K, et al. Functional anatomy of the posterolateral structures of the knee. Arthroscopy. 1993;9:57–62.
7. de Lima DA, et al. Anatomy of the anterolateral ligament of the knee: a systematic review. Arthroscopy. 2019;35:670–81.
8. Van Der Watt L, et al. The structure and function of the anterolateral ligament of the knee: a systematic review. Arthroscopy. 2015;31:569–582.e3.
9. Pomajzl R, Maerz T, Shams C, Guettler J, Bicos J. A review of the anterolateral ligament of the knee: current knowledge regarding its incidence, anatomy, biomechanics, and surgical dissection. Arthroscopy. 2015;31:583–91.
10. Claes S, et al. Anatomy of the anterolateral ligament of the knee. J Anat. 2013;223:321–8.
11. Vincent JP, et al. The anterolateral ligament of the human knee: an anatomic and histologic study. Knee Surg Sports Traumatol Arthrosc. 2012;20:147–52.
12. Irvine GB, Dias JJ, Finlay DBL. Segond fractures of the lateral tibial condyle: brief report. J Bone Joint Surg Br. 1987;69:613–4.

13. Campos JC, et al. Pathogenesis of the segond fracture: anatomic and MR imaging evidence of an iliotibial tract or anterior oblique band avulsion. Radiology. 2001;219:381–6.
14. Olewnik Ł, et al. The anterolateral ligament of the knee: a proposed classification system. Clin Anat. 2018;31:966–73.
15. Kraeutler MJ, Welton KL, Chahla J, LaPrade RF, McCarty EC. Current concepts of the anterolateral ligament of the knee: anatomy, biomechanics, and reconstruction. Am J Sports Med. 2018;46:1235–42.
16. Shetty A, et al. Lateral collateral ligament and anterolateral ligament of the knee—a morphological analysis with orthopedic significance. Knee. 2021;28:202–6.
17. Helito CP, et al. Anatomy and histology of the knee anterolateral ligament. Orthop J Sport Med. 2013;1:354.
18. Daggett M, Busch K, Sonnery-Cottet B. Surgical dissection of the anterolateral ligament. Arthrosc Tech. 2016;5:e185.
19. Ahn SJ, Jeong YM, Lee BG, et al. Using three-dimensional isotropic SPACE MRI to detect posterolateral corner injury of the knee. Acta Radiol. 2016;57(10):1251–60.
20. Gollehon DL, Torzilli PA, Warren RF. The role of the posterolateral and cruciate ligaments in the stability of the human knee: a biomechanical study. J Bone Joint Surg Am. 1987;69(2):233–42.
21. LaPrade RF, Ly TV, Wentorf FA, Engebretsen I. The posterolateral attachments of the knee: a qualitative and quantitative morphologic analysis of the fibular collateral ligament, popliteus tendon, popliteofibular ligament, and lateral gastrocnemius tendon. Am J Sports Med. 2003;31(6):854–60.
22. Veltri DM, Deng XH, Torzilli PA, Maynard MJ, Warren RF. The role of the popliteofibular ligament in stability of the human knee: a biomechanical study. Am J Sports Med. 1996;24(1):19–27.
23. De Maeseneer M, Shahabpour M, Vanderdood K, De Ridder F, Van Roy F, Osteaux M. Posterolateral supporting structures of the knee: findings on anatomic dissection, anatomic slices and MR images. Eur Radiol. 2001;11(11):2170–7.
24. LaPrade RF, Bollom TS, Wentorf FA, Wills NJ, Meister K. Mechanical properties of the posterolateral structures of the knee. Am J Sports Med. 2005;33(9):1386–91.
25. LaPrade RF, Gilbert TJ, Bollom TS, Wentorf F, Chaljub G. The magnetic resonance imaging appearance of individual structures of the posterolateral knee: a prospective study of normal knees and knees with surgically verified grade III injuries. Am J Sports Med. 2000;28(2):191–9.
26. LaPrade RF, Wentorf FA, Fritts H, Gundry C, Hightower CD. A prospective magnetic resonance imaging study of the incidence of posterolateral and multiple ligament injuries in acute knee injuries presenting with a hemarthrosis. Arthroscopy. 2007;23(12):1341–7.
27. Sekiya JK, Jacobson JA, Wojtys EM. Sonographic imaging of the posterolateral structures of the knee: findings in human cadavers. Arthroscopy. 2002;18(8):872–81.
28. McKean D, Yoong P, Yanny S, et al. The popliteal fibular ligament in acute knee trauma: patterns of injury on MR imaging. Skeletal Radiol. 2015;44(10):1413–9.
29. Bolog N, Hodler J. MR imaging of the posterolateral corner of the knee. Skeletal Radiol. 2007;36(8):715–28.
30. Huang G-S, Yu JS, Munshi M, et al. Avulsion fracture of the head of the fibula (the "arcuate" sign): MR imaging findings predictive of injuries to the posterolateral ligaments and posterior cruciate ligament. AJR Am J Roentgenol. 2003;180(2):381–7.
31. Pękala PA, Mann MR, Pękala JR, et al. The gastrocnemiofibular ligament: a new, more anatomically accurate name for the fabellofibular ligament—an original magnetic resonance imaging study and meta-analysis. Clin Anat. 2020;33(3):419–27.
32. Pękala PA, Mann MR, Pękala JR, Tomaszewski KA, LaPrade RF. Evidence-based clinical anatomy of the popliteofibular ligament and its importance in orthopaedic surgery. Am J Sports Med. 2020;5:363546520950415.

33. Sekiya JK, Swaringen JC, Wojtys EM, Jacobson JA. Diagnostic ultrasound evaluation of posterolateral corner knee injuries. Arthroscopy. 2010;26(4):494–9.
34. Gray H. Anatomy of the human body. 20th ed. Philadelphia: Lea & Febiger; 1918.
35. Ellis R, Hing W, Reid D. Iliotibial band friction syndrome—a systematic review. Man Ther. 2007;12(3):200–8.
36. Kaplan EB. The iliotibial tract; clinical and morphological significance. J Bone Joint Surg Am. 1958;40-A(4):817–32.
37. Huang BK, Campos JC, Michael Peschka PG, et al. Injury of the gluteal aponeurotic fascia and proximal iliotibial band: anatomy, pathologic conditions, and MR imaging. Radiographics. 2013;33(5):1437–52.
38. Cruells Vieira EL, et al. An anatomic study of the iliotibial tract. Arthroscopy. 2007;23:269–74.
39. Birnbaum K, Siebert CH, Pandorf T, Schopphoff E, Prescher A, Niethard FU. Anatomical and biomechanical investigations of the iliotibial tract. Surg Radiol Anat. 2004;26(6):433–46.
40. Hirschmann MT, Müller W. Complex function of the knee joint: the current understanding of the knee. Knee Surg Sports Traumatol Arthrosc. 2015;23(10):2780–8.
41. Terry GC, Hughston JC, Norwood LA. The anatomy of the iliopatellar band and iliotibial tract. Am J Sports Med. 1986;14:39–45.
42. Vinson EN, Major NM, Helms CA. The posterolateral corner of the knee. AJR Am J Roentgenol. 2008;190(2):449–58.
43. Mansour R, Yoong P, McKean D, Teh JL. The iliotibial band in acute knee trauma: patterns of injury on MR imaging. Skeletal Radiol. 2014;43(10):1369–75.
44. Murphy BJ, Hechtman KS, Uribe JW, Selesnick H, Smith RL, Zlatkin MB. Iliotibial band friction syndrome: MR imaging findings. Radiology. 1992;185(2):569–71.
45. Vasilevska V, Szeimies U, Stäbler A. Magnetic resonance imaging signs of iliotibial band friction in patients with isolated medial compartment osteoarthritis of the knee. Skeletal Radiol. 2009;38(9):871–5.
46. Muhle C, Ahn JM, Yeh L, et al. Iliotibial band friction syndrome: MR imaging findings in 16 patients and MR arthrographic study of six cadaveric knees. Radiology. 1999;212(1):103–10.
47. Ekman EF, Pope T, Martin DF, Curl WW. Magnetic resonance imaging of iliotibial band syndrome. Am J Sports Med. 1994;22(6):851–4.
48. De Maeseneer M, Marcelis S, Boulet C, et al. Ultrasound of the knee with emphasis on the detailed anatomy of anterior, medial, and lateral structures. Skeletal Radiol. 2014;43(8):1025–39.
49. Marchand AJ, Proisy M, Ropars M, Cohen M, Duvauferrier R, Guillin R. Snapping knee: imaging findings with an emphasis on dynamic sonography. AJR Am J Roentgenol. 2012;199(1):142–50.
50. Lewis CL. Extra-articular snapping hip: a literature review. Sports Health. 2010;2(3):186–90.
51. Pelsser V, Cardinal E, Hobden R, Aubin B, Lafortune M. Extraarticular snapping hip: sonographic findings. AJR Am J Roentgenol. 2001;176(1):67–73.
52. Sher I, Umans H, Downie SA, Tobin K, Arora R, Olson TR. Proximal iliotibial band syndrome: what is it and where is it? Skeletal Radiol. 2011;40(12):1553–6.
53. Bonilla-Yoon I, Masih S, Patel DB, et al. The Morel-Lavallée lesion: pathophysiology, clinical presentation, imaging features, and treatment options. Emerg Radiol. 2014;21(1):35–43.
54. Mellado JM, Bencardino JT. Morel-Lavallée lesion: review with emphasis on MR imaging. Magn Reson Imaging Clin N Am. 2005;13(4):775–82.
55. Choi YS, Lee SM, Song BY, Paik SH, Yoon YK. Dynamic sonography of external snapping hip syndrome. J Ultrasound Med. 2002;21(7):753–8.
56. Chang KS, Cheng YH, Wu CH, Özçakar L. Dynamic ultrasound imaging for the iliotibial band/snapping hip syndrome. Am J Phys Med Rehabil. 2015;94(6):e55–6.
57. Krishnamurthy G, Connolly BL, Narayanan U, Babyn PS. Imaging findings in external snapping hip syndrome. Pediatr Radiol. 2007;37(12):1272–4.

58. Chang CY, Kreher J, Torriani M. Dynamic sonography of snapping hip due to gluteus maximus subluxation over greater trochanter. Skeletal Radiol. 2016;45(3):409–12.
59. Zbojniewicz AM. US for diagnosis of musculoskeletal conditions in the young athlete: emphasis on dynamic assessment. Radiographics. 2014;34(5):1145–62.
60. Deslandes M, Guillin R, Cardinal E, Hobden R, Bureau NJ. The snapping iliopsoas tendon: new mechanisms using dynamic sonography. AJR Am J Roentgenol. 2008;190(3):576–81.
61. Isusi M, Oleaga L, Campo M, Grande D. MRI findings in iliotibial band friction syndrome: a report of two cases. Radiologia. 2007;49(6):433–5.
62. Grando H, Chang EY, Chen KC, Chung CB. MR imaging of extrasynovial inflammation and impingement about the knee. Magn Reson Imaging Clin N Am. 2014;22(4):725–41.
63. Terry GC, Norwood LA, Hughston JC, Caldwell KM. How iliotibial tract injuries of the knee combine with acute anterior cruciate ligament tears to influence abnormal anterior tibial displacement. Am J Sports Med. 1993;21(1):55–60.
64. Arend CF. Sonography of the iliotibial band: spectrum of findings. Radiol Bras. 2014;47:33–7.
65. Haims AH, Medvecky MJ, Pavlovich R, Katz LD. MR imaging of the anatomy of and injuries to the lateral and posterolateral aspects of the knee. AJR Am J Roentgenol. 2003;180(3):647–53.
66. Gottsegen CJ, Eyer BA, White EA, Learch TJ, Forrester D. Avulsion fractures of the knee: imaging findings and clinical significance. Radiographics. 2008;28(6):1755–70.
67. Fay K, Mannem R, Baynes K, Sarin D, DuBois M. Iliotibial band avulsion fracture: a case report with differential diagnosis. Emerg Radiol. 2016;23(1):93–6.
68. Yoo JH, Hahn SH, Yang BK, et al. An en bloc avulsion fracture of tibial tuberosity and Gerdy's tubercle in an adolescent basketball player: a case report. Knee Surg Sports Traumatol Arthrosc. 2007;15(6):781–5.
69. Helito CP, Helito PV, Bonadio MB, et al. Correlation of magnetic resonance imaging with knee anterolateral ligament anatomy: a cadaveric study. Orthop J Sports Med. 2015;3(12):2325967115621024.
70. Van Dyck P, Clockaerts S, Vanhoenacker FM, et al. Anterolateral ligament abnormalities in patients with acute anterior cruciate ligament rupture are associated with lateral meniscal and osseous injuries. Eur Radiol. 2016;26(10):3383–91.
71. Weber WN, Neumann CH, Barakos JA, Petersen SA, Steinbach LS, Genant HK. Lateral tibial rim (Segond) fractures: MR imaging characteristics. Radiology. 1991;180(3):731–4.
72. Porrino J Jr, Maloney E, Richardson M, Mulcahy H, Ha A, Chew FS. The anterolateral ligament of the knee: MRI appearance, association with the Segond fracture, and historical perspective. AJR Am J Roentgenol. 2015;204(2):367–73.
73. Helito CP, Helito PV, Costa HP, et al. MRI evaluation of the anterolateral ligament of the knee: assessment in routine 1.5-T scans. Skeletal Radiol. 2014;43(10):1421–7.
74. Morgan PM, LaPrade RF, Wentorf FA, Cook JW, Bianco A. The role of the oblique popliteal ligament and other structures in preventing knee hyperextension. Am J Sports Med. 2010;38:550–7. https://doi.org/10.1177/0363546509348742.
75. Standring S. Gray's anatomy: The anatomical basis of clinical practice. 41st ed. London: Elsevier Health Sciences; 2016. p. 114, 1366, 1398.
76. Scapinelli R. Vascular anatomy of the human cruciate ligaments and surrounding structures. Clin Anat. 1997;10:151–62. https://doi.org/10.1002/(SICI)1098-2353(1997)10:3<151::AID-CA1>3.0.CO;2-X.
77. Schunke M, Schulte E, Schumacher U, Rude J, Voll MM, Wesler K. Thieme atlas of anatomy: general anatomy and musculoskeletal system. New York: Thieme, Stuttgart; 2006. p. 501.
78. Bozkurt M, Elhan A, Tekdemir I, Tonuk E. An anatomical study of the meniscofibular ligament. Knee Surg Sports Traumatol Arthrosc. 2004;12:429–33. https://doi.org/10.1007/s00167-003-0450-z.
79. Natsis K, Paraskevas G, Anastasopoulos N, et al. Meniscofibular ligament: morphology and functional significance of a relatively unknown anatomical structure. Anat Res Int. 2012;2012:214784. https://doi.org/10.1155/2012/214784.

80. Covey DC. Injuries of the posterolateral corner of the knee. J Bone Joint Surg Am. 2001;83:106–18. https://doi.org/10.2106/00004623-200101000-00015.
81. Obaid H, Gartner L, Haydar AA, et al. The meniscofibular ligament: an MRI study. Eur J Radiol. 2010;73:159–61. https://doi.org/10.1016/j.ejrad.2008.09.026.
82. Vap AR, Schon JM, Moatshe G, et al. The role of the peripheral passive rotation stabilizers of the knee with intact collateral and cruciate ligaments: a biomechanical study. Orthop J Sport Med. 2017;5:2325967117708190. https://doi.org/10.1177/2325967117708190.
83. Unay K, Ozkan K, Esenkaya I, et al. Rupture of the meniscofibular ligament. J Orthop Surg Res. 2010;5:35. https://doi.org/10.1186/1749-799X-5-35.
84. LaPrade RF, Morgan PM, Wentorf FA, Johansen S, Engebretsen L. The anatomy of the posterior aspect of the knee. An anatomic study. J Bone Joint Surg Am. 2007;89:758–64. https://doi.org/10.2106/JBJS.F.00120.
85. Osti M, Tschann P, Künzel KH, Benedetto KP. Posterolateral corner of the knee: microsurgical analysis of anatomy and morphometry. Orthopedics. 2013;36(9):e1114–20. https://doi.org/10.3928/01477447-20130821-11.
86. Wu XD, Yu JH, Zou T, Wang W, LaPrade RF, Huang W, Sun SQ. Anatomical characteristics and biomechanical properties of the oblique popliteal ligament. Sci Rep. 2017;16(7):42698. https://doi.org/10.1038/srep42698.
87. LaPrade RF, Morgan PM, Wentorf FA, Johansen S, Engebretsen L. The anatomy of the posterior aspect of the knee. An anatomic study. J Bone Joint Surg Am. 2007;89:758–64.
88. Fam LPD, Fruheling VM, Pupim B, Ramos CH, de Moura MFA, Namba M, da Silva JLV, da Cunha LAM, de Oliveira Franco APG, Filho ES. Oblique popliteal ligament—an anatomical study. Rev Bras Ortop. 2013;48(5):402–5. https://doi.org/10.1016/j.rboe.2012.07.010.
89. Hedderwick M. The anatomy of the oblique popliteal ligament (Thesis, Master of Science). University of Otago. Available at: http://hdl.handle.net/10523/2359 (2012).
90. Margareta N, Victor HF. Basic biomechanics of the musculoskeletal system. 3rd ed. Philadelphia: Lippincott Williams & Wilkins; 2001.
91. Shoemaker SC, Markolf KL. In vivo rotatory knee stability. Ligamentous and muscular contributions. J Bone Joint Surg Am. 1982;64:208–16.
92. Wang CJ, Walker PS. Rotatory laxity of the human knee joint. J Bone Joint Surg Am. 1974;56:161–70.
93. Matsumoto H, Seedhom BB, Suda Y, Otani T, Fujikawa K. Axis location of tibial rotation and its change with flexion angle. Clin Orthop Relat Res. 2000;371:178–82.
94. Dannawi Z, Khanduja V, Vemulapalli K. Arthroscopic excision of the fabella. J Knee Surg. 2007;20:299–301.
95. Franceschi F, Longo UG, Ruzzini L, Leonardi F, Rojas M, Gualdi G, Denaro V. Dislocation of an enlarged fabella as uncommon cause of knee pain: a case report. Knee. 2007;14:330–2.
96. Kawashima T, Takeishi H, Yoshitomi S, Ito M, Sasaki H. Anatomical study of the fabella, fabellar complex and its clinical implications. Surg Radiol Anat. 2007;29:611–6. https://doi.org/10.1007/s00276-007-0259-4.
97. Minowa T, Murakami G, Kura H, Suzuki D, Han SH, Yamashita T. Does the fabella contribute to the reinforcement of the posterolateral corner of the knee by inducing the development of associated ligaments? J Orthop Sci. 2004;9:59–65.
98. Last RJ. The popliteus muscle and the lateral meniscus. J Bone Joint Surg (Br). 1950;32:93–9.
99. Staubli HU, Birrer S. The popliteus muscle and its fascicles at the popliteal hiatus: gross anatomy and functional arthroscopic evaluation. Arthroscopy. 1990;6:209–20.
100. Covey DC. Current concepts review: injuries of the posterolateral corner of the knee. J Bone Joint Surg Am. 2001;83:106–18.
101. Watanabe Y, Moriya H, Takahashi K. Functional anatomy of the posterolateral structures of the knee. Arthroscopy. 1993;9:460–2.
102. Seebacher JR, Inglis AE, Marshall JL, Warren RF. The structure of the posterolateral aspect of the knee. J Bone Joint Surg Am. 1982;64:536–42.

103. Shahane SA, Ibbotson C, Strachan R, Bickerstaff DR. The popliteofibular ligament: an anatomic study of the posterolateral corner of the knee. J Bone Joint Surg (Br). 1999;81:636–42.
104. Johnson ME, Foster L, DeLee JC. Neurologic and vascular injuries associated with knee ligament injuries. Am J Sports Med. 2008;36:2448–62. https://doi.org/10.1177/0363546508325669.
105. Khan R, Birch R. Latropathic injuries of peripheral nerves. J Bone Joint Surg Br. 2001;83:1145–8.
106. Kim DH, Murovic JA, Tiel RL, Kline DG. Management and outcomes in 318 operative common peroneal nerve lesions at the Louisiana State University Health Sciences Center. Neurosurgery. 2004;54:1421–8.
107. Stufkens SA, van den Bekerom MPJ, Doornberg JN, et al. Evidence-based treatment of maisonneuve fractures. J Foot Ankle Surg. 2011;50:62–7. https://doi.org/10.1053/j.jfas.2010.08.017.
108. Stitgen SH, Cairns ER, Ebraheim N, et al. Anatomic considerations of pin placement in the proximal tibia and its relationship to the peroneal nerve. Clin Orthop Relat Res. 1992;278:134–7.
109. Rubel IF, Schwarzbard I, Leonard A, Cece D. Anatomic location of the peroneal nerve at the level of the proximal aspect of the tibia: Gerdy's safe zone. J Bone Joint Surg Am. 2004;86-A:1625–8.
110. Takeda A, Tsucbiya H, Mori Y, et al. Anatomical aspects of biopsy of the proximal fibula. Int Orthop. 2001;24:335–7. https://doi.org/10.1007/s002640000185.
111. Hildebrand G, Tompkins M, Macalena J. Fibular head as a landmark for identification of the common peroneal nerve: a cadaveric study. Arthrosc J Arthrosc Relat Surg. 2015;31:99–103. https://doi.org/10.1016/j.arthro.2014.07.014.
112. Ryan W, Mahony N, Delaney M, et al. Relationship of the common peroneal nerve and its branches to the head and neck of the fibula. Clin Anat. 2003;16:501–5. https://doi.org/10.1002/ca.10155.
113. Mendes E, da Silva MV. Anatomy of the lateral collateral ligament: a cadaver and histological study. Knee Surg Sports Traumatol Arthrosc. 2005; https://doi.org/10.1007/s00167-005-0681-2.
114. Kumar A, Raza K, Krishna H, Narayan RK, Jha RK, Kumari C, Asghar A, Kumar T, Agrawal P. Sharing of proximal fibers by the anterolateral and lateral collateral ligaments in the human knee: a cadaveric study. Sci Rep. 2023; https://doi.org/10.1038/s41598-023-38211-9.
115. Pękala PA, Mizia E, Mann MR, Wagner-Olszewska I, Mostowy M, Tatoń G, Domżalski M. The popliteofibular ligament: a cadaveric ultrasound study. Skeletal Radiol. 2021; https://doi.org/10.1007/s00256-021-03813-9.
116. Flato R, Passanante GJ, Skalski MR, Patel DB, White EA, Matcuk GR. The iliotibial tract: imaging, anatomy, injuries, and other pathology. Skeletal Radiol. 2017; https://doi.org/10.1007/s00256-017-2604-y.
117. Hedderwick M, Stringer MD, McRedmond L, Meikle GR, Woodley SJ. The oblique popliteal ligament: an anatomic and MRI investigation. Surg Radiol Anat. 2017; https://doi.org/10.1007/s00276-017-1838-7.
118. Natsis K, Karasavvidis T, Kola D, Papadopoulos S, Totlis T. Meniscofibular ligament: how much do we know about this structure of the posterolateral corner of the knee: anatomical study and review of literature. Surg Radiol Anat. 2020; https://doi.org/10.1007/s00276-020-02459-x.
119. Kancharla E, Jeph RB, Ravichandran S, Mehta V, Loh HK. Morphological and morphometric analysis of oblique popliteal ligament in North Indian population: a cadaveric study. Surg Radiol Anat. 2024; https://doi.org/10.1007/s00276-023-03288-4.
120. Wu X-D, Yu J-H, Zou T, Wang W, LaPrade RF, Huang W, Sun S-Q. Anatomical characteristics and biomechanical properties of the oblique popliteal ligament. Sci Rep. 2017; https://doi.org/10.1038/srep42698.

121. Zeng S-X, Dong X-L, Dang R-S, Wu G-S, Wang J-F, Wang D, Huang H-L, Guo X-D. Anatomic study of fabella and its surrounding structures in a Chinese population. Surg Radiol Anat. 2011; https://doi.org/10.1007/s00276-011-0828-4.
122. Wadia FD, Pimple M, Gajjar SM, Narvekar AD. An anatomic study of the popliteofibular ligament. Int Orthop. 2003; https://doi.org/10.1007/s00264-003-0445-x.
123. Rausch V, Hackl M, Oppermann J, Leschinger T, Scaal M, Müller LP, Wegmann K. Peroneal nerve location at the fibular head: an anatomic study using 3D imaging. Arch Orthop Trauma Surg. 2019; https://doi.org/10.1007/s00402-019-03141-7.

Part II
Surfaces of the Knee

1.1 Introduction by the Editor

The surfaces of the knee interact with the ligaments to guide the joint through a complex range of motion. The femoral condyles are asymmetric and articulate with a concave medial tibial plateau and a convex lateral tibial plateau surface. The patella has seven facets that articulate with the trochlea of the femur and increases the mechanical advantage of the quadriceps mechanism.

Chapter 5
The Femoral Anatomy

Alfred J. Tria Jr. and Giles R. Scuderi

Machine Generated Summaries

Disclaimer: The summaries in this chapter were generated from Springer Nature publications using abstractive AI auto-summarization: An abstraction-based summarizer creates new text based on deep learning. New phrases are created to summarize the content. As the constituted sentences are machine selected, they may not fully reflect the body of the work, so we strongly advise that the original content is read and cited. The auto-generated summaries were curated by the editor to meet Springer Nature publication standards.

Machine generated keywords: notch, intercondylar notch, intercondylar, acl, roof, canal, nutrient, meniscus, height width, ctlinr, meniscus tear, artery, nutrient artery, femur height, artery canal.

Femoral Intercondylar Notch: Gross Anatomy and Histology of the Connective Tissue Lining of Its Roof: A Pilot Study [57]

This is a machine-generated summary of:

Nag, Hira Lal; Jain, Gunjar; Vijayakumar, Vivek; Jacob, Tony George; Sonai, Mukinkumar; Lalwani, Sanjeev: Femoral Intercondylar Notch: Gross Anatomy and Histology of the Connective Tissue Lining of its Roof: A Pilot Study [57]

Published in: Surgical and Radiologic Anatomy (2021)

A. J. Tria Jr. (✉)
Department of Orthopedics, Rutgers-Robert Wood Johnson Medical School, New Brunswick, NJ, USA

G. R. Scuderi
Northwell Health Orthopaedic Institute, New York, NY, USA

A. J. Tria Jr., G. R. Scuderi (eds.), *Ligaments of the Knee*, https://doi.org/10.1007/978-3-031-66615-5_5

Link to original: https://doi.org/10.1007/s00276-021-02757-y

If you want to cite the papers, please refer to the original.
For technical reasons we could not place the page where the original quote is coming from.

Research Highlights
The intercondylar notch of the distal femur, a key structure in knee joint mechanics, is lined with a connective tissue that has been routinely observed during arthroscopic surgeries. This lining's relationship with the anterior cruciate ligament (ACL) is crucial, as variations in its morphology can influence ACL injury risk and post-surgical outcomes. Nag et al. addresses a significant knowledge gap by investigating the anatomy of the connective tissue lining of the intercondylar notch's roof (CTLINR), a structure whose detailed anatomical and radiological characteristics have not been previously described.

Nag utilized cadaveric specimens to conduct an observational anatomical study, dissecting the knees to examine the CTLINR's gross anatomical features and its relationship with the cruciate ligaments. They preserved and analyzed tissue samples, complementing their findings with histological examinations. The authors suggest that this connective tissue may play a protective role for the ACL, The study faced limitations due to post-mortem degradation, which necessitated obtaining additional tissue from a living patient for electron microscopy analysis. Despite these challenges, Nag characterized the CTLINR's appearance, texture, and cellular composition.

This study marks an advance in our understanding of knee joint anatomy by identifying and describing the CTLINR as a distinct anatomical entity. The researchers found that this tissue is not only structurally different from the ACL but also appears to serve as a protective layer. This research opens up new avenues for investigating how this structure could be preserved during ACL reconstruction to potentially improve surgical outcomes. While further research is needed to fully understand its physiological function and implications for surgical practice, this preliminary study lays the groundwork for future investigations into the CTLINR's role in knee joint health and injury prevention.

Is There Any Relation Between Distal Parameters of the Femur and Its Height and Width? [58]

This is a machine-generated summary of:

Yazar, Fatih; Imre, Nurcan; Battal, Bilal; Bilgic, Serkan; Tayfun, Cem: Is there any relation between distal parameters of the femur and its height and width? [58]

Published in: Surgical and Radiologic Anatomy (2011)
Link to original: https://doi.org/10.1007/s00276-011-0847-1

If you want to cite the papers, please refer to the original.

For technical reasons we could not place the page where the original quote is coming from.

Research Highlights

The intricate morphology of the distal femur plays a crucial role in knee joint stability and is a key consideration in total knee arthroplasty. Despite its importance, current anatomical descriptions of the distal femoral epicondyles remain imprecise, leading to challenges in prosthesis design and fit, particularly across diverse populations. Yazar et al. addresses this gap by investigating the morphometry of the distal femur and its relationship with femoral height and width, providing insights that could assist in prosthesis selection and manufacturing.

Yazar utilized sixty-six adult Caucasian dry femurs for the analysis, employing computer tomography (CT) imaging to ensure precise measurements. The authors measured various parameters of the distal femur, including medial-lateral intercondylar distances at different sections, to derive an average value for each dimension. Statistical analyses were performed using SPSS software, with significance set at $p < 0.05$. The study found significant correlations between femur height and width with other measured parameters, suggesting that these two dimensions could be pivotal in determining prosthesis size.

The findings of this study represent a significant advance in our understanding of distal femur morphology and its implications for knee arthroplasty. The results indicate that simply knowing the measures of femur height and width can be the main factor in determining prosthesis selection, emphasizing the practical applications of their findings. By demonstrating strong correlations between these measurements and other morphometric parameters, the study suggests that individual anthropometry should guide prosthesis design rather than relying on population averages or gender distinctions. Looking ahead, this research paves the way for more personalized approaches to knee arthroplasty.

Distal Femur Morphometry: A Gender and Bilateral Comparative Study Using Magnetic Resonance Imaging [59]

This is a machine-generated summary of:

Murshed, Khalil Awadh; Çiçekcibaşi, Aynur Emine; Karabacakoğlu, Aydın; Şeker, Muzaffer; Ziylan, Taner: Distal femur morphometry: a gender and bilateral comparative study using magnetic resonance imaging [59]

Published in: Surgical and Radiologic Anatomy (2004)

Link to original: https://doi.org/10.1007/s00276-004-0295-2

If you want to cite the papers, please refer to the original.

For technical reasons we could not place the page where the original quote is coming from.

Research Highlights

The intercondylar notch of the knee plays a critical role in the health and integrity of the anterior cruciate ligament (ACL), with its dimensions being a key factor in assessing ACL injury risk and surgical outcomes. Despite its clinical importance, there is a lack of consensus on how notch dimensions vary between genders and how this might contribute to ACL injury susceptibility. Murshed et al. has sought to clarify these uncertainties by examining the intercondylar notch size index (NSI) across male and female MRI samples, providing insights into the anatomical differences that may influence ACL injuries.

Murshed analyzed 200 knee axial MRI examinations from the Radiology Department of Meram Faculty of Medicine at Selçuk University. The subjects, ranging in age from 18 to 65 years, were selected for having no morphologic knee abnormalities. Using a 1.5 T superconducting unit with T1-weighted axial images, the team measured various parameters including the maximal height and transverse width of the intercondylar notch, epicondylar width, and lateral condylar width. The NSI was calculated by dividing the notch width by its height.,capturing a detailed picture of the intercondylar notch geometry.

Statistical analysis using SPSS revealed significant gender differences in several measurements, with males generally exhibiting larger dimensions than females. However, no significant difference was found in NSI between genders. Age showed an inversely significant correlation with all measurements, suggesting that notch dimensions decrease with age.

This study represents a significant advance in our understanding of knee anatomy and its implications for ACL injury risk. By demonstrating that while there are clear gender differences in certain aspects of knee morphology, these do not necessarily translate to differences in NSI, Murshed challenges some prevailing assumptions about gender-specific risk factors for ACL injuries. Their findings underscore the complexity of factors contributing to ACL injuries and may have important implications for both diagnosis and treatment. Looking forward, this research paves the way for more personalized approaches to ACL injury prevention and management, taking into account individual anatomical variations rather than relying on broad gender-based assumptions.

The Potential Effect of Anatomic Relationship Between the Femur and the Tibia on Medial Meniscus Tears [60]

This is a machine-generated summary of:

Bozkurt, Murat; Unlu, Serhan; Cay, Nurdan; Apaydin, Nihal; Dogan, Metin: The potential effect of anatomic relationship between the femur and the tibia on medial meniscus tears [60]

Published in: Surgical and Radiologic Anatomy (2014)

Link to original: https://doi.org/10.1007/s00276-014-1266-x

If you want to cite the papers, please refer to the original.

For technical reasons we could not place the page where the original quote is coming from.

Research Highlights

Understanding the intricate relationship between knee morphology and kinematics is crucial for addressing various knee pathologies. While previous research has established the circular nature of posterior femoral condyles and their role in tracking femorotibial movement, the impact of morphometric incongruence on meniscal lesions remains underexplored. Bozkurt et al. aims to bridge this knowledge gap by evaluating the influence of femorotibial incongruence on both medial and lateral meniscus tears.

Bozkurt conducted an investigation using MRI scans from two radiology centers, ensuring no confounding injuries or surgeries could skew results. The scans underwent analysis with Materialise's Interactive Medical Image Control System, with repeated measurements to minimize observer variability. Statistical tools like SPSS software provided robust data analysis, revealing significant correlations between the diameters of femoral condyles, tibial articular surfaces, and meniscus tears.

The study demonstrated that femorotibial incongruence significantly correlates with medial meniscus tears, suggesting that morphometric characteristics are not just a detail but a determinant in knee health. This insight opens avenues for tailored treatment plans and preventative strategies against osteoarthritis and other degenerative conditions. This study highlights, addressing the nuances of knee morphology could be key to improving clinical outcomes for patients suffering from meniscal injuries.

The Demonstration of the Number, Course, and the Location of Nutrient Artery Canals of the Femur by Multidetector Computed Tomography [61]

This is a machine-generated summary of:

Imre, Nurcan; Battal, Bilal; Acikel, Cengiz Han; Akgun, Veysel; Comert, Ayhan; Yazar, Fatih: The demonstration of the number, course, and the location of nutrient artery canals of the femur by multidetector computed tomography [61]

Published in: Surgical and Radiologic Anatomy (2012)

Link to original: https://doi.org/10.1007/s00276-011-0930-7

If you want to cite the papers, please refer to the original.

For technical reasons we could not place the page where the original quote is coming from.

Research Highlights

Understanding the vascular anatomy of long bones is crucial for surgical interventions and treatment of bone pathologies. The femur, with its complex circulatory systems including the nutritional system, metaphyseal complex, and periosteal capillary system, relies heavily on nutrient arteries for blood supply. However, the precise mapping of these nutrient artery canals in the femur has been limited by traditional observation methods. Imre et al. employed multidetector computed tomography (MDCT) to evaluate the number, courses, widths, and locations of nutrient artery canals in the femur with unprecedented detail.

Imre analyzed sixty-six adult dry femurs using MDCT, which allows for high-resolution imaging and detailed three-dimensional reconstructions. This advanced imaging technique surpasses previous methods by enabling visualization of both external and internal features of nutrient artery canals. The arterial canals were identified based on specific criteria such as an uninterrupted cortical course and an inner ostium opening to the medullary cavity. The authors classified these canals by their orientation and segmental location along the femur. Statistical analysis revealed patterns in canal dimensions and correlations between canal numbers and diameters.

The findings significantly enhance our understanding of femoral vascular anatomy. Most notably, it was discovered that the majority of nutrient artery canals are located in the middle segment of the femur and predominantly enter through or near the linea aspera. The research also suggests that while canal diameters tend to decrease with an increasing number of canals, there is no significant variation in diameter based on their position relative to the linea aspera or along different segments of the bone. These insights have immediate clinical implications; recognizing canal locations could prevent inadvertent damage during surgery. Looking forward, this study sets a new standard for anatomical studies using MDCT and paves the way for further research into how these vascular channels influence bone growth and healing processes.

Bibliography

1. Stäubli HU, Rauschning W. Tibial attachment area of the anterior cruciate ligament in the extended knee position. Knee Surg Sports Traumatol Arthrosc. 1994;2(3):138–46.
2. Huang M, Li Y, Guo N, Liao C, Yu B. Relationship between intercondylar notch angle and anterior cruciate ligament injury: a magnetic resonance imaging analysis. J Int Med Res. 2019;47(4):1602–9.
3. Samora W, Beran MC, Parikh SN. Intercondylar roof inclination angle: is it a risk factor for ACL tears or tibial spine fractures? J Pediatr Orthop. 2016;36(6):e71–4.
4. Scheffel PT, Henninger HB, Burks RT. Relationship of the intercondylar roof and the tibial footprint of the ACL: implications for ACL reconstruction. Am J Sports Med. 2013;41(2):396–401.
5. Cha JH, Lee SH, Shin MJ, Choi BK, Bin SI. Relationship between mucoid hypertrophy of the anterior cruciate ligament (ACL) and morphologic change of the intercondylar notch: MRI and arthroscopy correlation. Skeletal Radiol. 2008;37(9):821–6.
6. Li H, Zeng C, Wang Y, Wei J, Yang T, Cui Y, Xie D, Liu H, Lei GH. Association between magnetic resonance imaging-measured intercondylar notch dimensions and anterior cruciate ligament injury: a meta-analysis. Arthroscopy. 2018;34(3):889–900.
7. Muneta T, Takakuda K, Yamamoto H. Intercondylar notch width and its relation to the configuration and cross-sectional area of the anterior cruciate ligament. A cadaveric knee study. Am J Sports Med. 1997;25(1):69–72.
8. Zeng C, Gao SG, Wei J, Yang TB, Cheng L, Luo W, Tu M, Xie Q, Hu Z, Liu PF, Li H, Yang T, Zhou B, Lei GH. The influence of the intercondylar notch dimensions on injury of the anterior cruciate ligament: a meta-analysis. Knee Surg Sports Traumatol Arthrosc. 2013;21(4):804–15.
9. Fung DT, Zhang LQ. Modeling of ACL impingement against the intercondylar notch. Clin Biomech. 2003;18(10):933–41.
10. Wilson R, Barhorst AA. Intercondylar notch impingement of the anterior cruciate ligament: a cadaveric in vitro study using robots. J Healthc Eng. 2018;10:1–27.
11. Pittner S, Monticelli FC, Pfisterer A, Zissler A, Sanger AM, Stoiber W, Steinbacher P. Postmortem degradation of skeletal muscle proteins: a novel approach to determine the time since death. Int J Legal Med. 2016;130(2):421–31.
12. Luetkemeyer CM, Marchi BC, Ashton-Miller JA, Arruda EM. Femoral entheseal shape and attachment angle as potential risk factors for anterior cruciate ligament injury. J Mech Behav Biomed Mater. 2018;88:313–21.
13. Śmigielski R, Zdanowicz U, Drwięga M, Ciszek B, Williams A. The anatomy of the anterior cruciate ligament and its relevance to the technique of reconstruction. Bone Joint J. 2016;98(8):1020–6.
14. Standring S, Gray H. Gray's anatomy. 40th ed. New York: Churchill Livingstone; 2008. p. 85.
15. Incavo SJ, Ronchetti PJ, Howe JG, Tranowski JP. Tibial plateau coverage in total knee arthroplasty. Clin Orthop Relat Res. 1994;299:81–5.
16. Westrich GH, Haas SB, Insall JN, Frachie A. Resection specimen analysis of proximal tibial anatomy based on 100 total knee arthroplasty specimens. J Arthroplast. 1995;10:47–51.
17. Cheng FB, Ji XF, Lai Y, et al. Three dimensional morphometry of the knee to design the total knee arthroplasty for Chinese population. Knee. 2009;16:341–7.
18. Dixon DR, Morgan R, Hollender LG, Roberts FA, O'Neal RB. Clinical application of spiral tomography in anterior implant placement: case report. J Periodontol. 2002;73:1202–9.

19. Lee IS, Choi JA, Kim TK, Han I, Lee JW, Kang HS. Reliability analysis of 16-MDCT in preoperative evaluation of total knee arthroplasty and comparison with intraoperative measurements. Am J Roentgenol. 2006;186:1778–82.
20. Uslu M, Ozsar B, Kendi T, Kara S, Tekdemir I, Atik OS. The use of computed tomography to determine femoral component size: a study of cadaver femora. Bull Hosp Joint Dis. 2005;63:49–53.
21. Low FH, Khoo LP, Chua CK, Lo NN. Determination of the major dimensions of femoral implants using morphometrical data and principal component analysis. Proc Inst Mech Eng H. 2000;214:301–9.
22. Wang SW, Feng CH, Lu HS. A study of Chinese knee joint geometry for prosthesis design. Chin Med J. 1992;105:227–33.
23. Yoshioka Y, Siu D, Cooke TDV. The anatomy and functional axes of the femur. J Bone Joint Surg. 1987;69:873–80.
24. Good L, Odensten M, Gillquist J. Intercondylar notch measurements with special reference to anterior cruciate ligament surgery. Clin Orthop. 1991;263:185–9.
25. Houseworth SW, Mauro VJ, Mellon BA, et al. The intercondylar notch in acute tears of the anterior cruciate ligament: a computer graphics study. Am J Sports Med. 1987;15:221–4.
26. Lund-Hanssen H, Gannon J, Engebretsen L, et al. Intercondylar notch width and the risk of anterior cruciate ligament rupture: a case control study in 46 female handball players. Acta Orthop Scand. 1994;65:529–32.
27. Ziylan T, Murshid KA. An analysis of Anatolian human femur anthropometry. Turk J Med Sci. 2002;32:231–5.
28. Kieffer DA, Curnow RJ, Southwell RB, et al. Anterior cruciate ligament arthroplasty. Am J Sports Med. 1984;12:301–12.
29. LaPrade RF, Burnett QM. Femoral intercondylar notch stenosis and correlation to anterior cruciate ligament injuries: a prospective study. Am J Sports Med. 1994;22:198–202.
30. Souryal TO, Moore HA, Evans JP. Bilaterality in anterior cruciate ligament injuries: associated intercondylar notch stenosis. Am J Sports Med. 1988;16:449–54.
31. Feagin JA Jr, Cabaud HE, Curl WW. The anterior cruciate ligament: radiographic and clinical signs of successful and unsuccessful repairs. Clin Orthop. 1982;164:54–8.
32. Odensten M, Gillquist J. Functional anatomy of the anterior cruciate ligament and a rationale for reconstruction. J Bone Joint Surg Am. 1985;67:257–62.
33. Koukoubis TD, Glisson RR, Bolognesi M, et al. Dimensions of the intercondylar notch of the knee. Am J Knee Surg. 1997;10:83–8.
34. Souryal TO, Freeman TR. Intercondylar notch size in anterior cruciate ligament injuries in athletes. A prospective study. Am J Sports Med. 1993;21:535–9.
35. Anderson AF, Dome DC, Gautam S, et al. Correlation of anthropometric measurements, strength, anterior cruciate ligament size, and intercondylar notch characteristics to sex differences in anterior cruciate ligament tear rates. Am J Sports Med. 2001;29:58–66.
36. Arendt E, Dick R. Knee injury patterns among men and women in collegiate basketball and soccer. NCAA data and review of literature. Am J Sports Med. 1995;23:694–701.
37. Clarke KS, Buckley WE. Women's injuries in collegiate sports. A preliminary comparative overview of three seasons. Am J Sports Med. 1980;8:187–91.
38. Engström B, Johansson C, Törnkvist H. Soccer injuries among elite female players. Am J Sports Med. 1991;19:372–5.
39. Ferretti A, Papandrea P, Conteduca F, et al. Knee ligament injuries in volleyball players. Am J Sports Med. 1992;20:203–7.
40. Gray J, Taunton JE, McKenzie DC, et al. A survey of injuries to the anterior cruciate ligament of the knee in female basketball players. Int J Sports Med. 1985;6:314–6.
41. Gwinn DE, Wilckens JH, McDevitt ER, et al. The relative incidence of anterior cruciate ligament injury in men and women at the United States Naval Academy. Am J Sports Med. 2000;28:98–102.

42. Ireland ML, Wall C. Epidemiology and comparison of knee injuries in elite male and female United States basketball athletes. Med Sci Sports Exerc. 1990;22:82.
43. Lindenfeld TN, Schmitt DJ, Hendy MP, et al. Incidence of injury in indoor soccer. Am J Sports Med. 1994;22:364–71.
44. Malone TR, Hardaker WT, Garrett WE, et al. Relationship of gender to anterior cruciate ligament injuries in intercollegiate basketball players. J South Orthop Assoc. 1993;2:36–9.
45. Zelisko JA, Noble HB, Porter M. A comparison of men's and women's professional basketball injuries. Am J Sports Med. 1982;10:297–9.
46. Zillmer DA, Powell JW, Albright JP. Gender-specific injury patterns in high school varsity basketball. J Women's Health. 1992;1:69–76.
47. Suganuma J. Lack of posteromedial tibiofemoral congruence at full flexion as a causative factor in isolated medial meniscal tears. J Orthop Sci. 2002;7:217–25.
48. Suganuma J, Mochizuki R, Yamaguchi K, Inoue Y, Yamabe E, Ueda Y, Fujinaka T. Cam impingement of the posterior femoral condyle in medial meniscal tears. Arthroscopy. 2010;26:173–83.
49. Bostrom M, Yang X, Koutras I. Biologics in bone healing. Curr Opin Orthop. 2000;11:403–12.
50. McKee NH, Haw P, Vettese T. Anatomic study of the nutrient foramen in the shaft of the fibula. Clin Orthop Rel Res. 1984;184:141–4.
51. Taylor GI. Fibular transplantation. In: Sefarin D, Burke HJ, editors. Microsurgical composite tissue transplantation. St Louis: Mosby; 1979. p. 418–23.
52. Gumusburun E, Yucel F, Ozkan Y, Akgun Z. A study of the nutrient foramina of lower limb long bones. Surg Radiol Anat. 1994;16:409–12.
53. Kizilkanat E, Boyan N, Ozsahin ET, Soames R, Oguz O. Location, number and clinical significance of nutrient foramina in human long bones. Ann Anat. 2007;189:87–95.
54. Schiessel A, Zweymüller K. The nutrient artery canal of the femur: a radiological study in patients with primary total hip replacement. Skel Radiol. 2004;33:142–9.
55. Bridgeman G, Brookes M. Blood supply to the human femoral diaphysis in youth and senescence. J Anat. 1996;188:611–21.
56. Lexer E, Kuligan P, Turk W. Untersuchungen über Knochenarterien. Berlin: Hirschwald; 1904.
57. Nag HL, Jain G, Vijayakumar V, Jacob TG, Sonai M, Lalwani S. Femoral intercondylar notch: gross anatomy and histology of the connective tissue lining of its roof: a pilot study. Surg Radiol Anat. 2021; https://doi.org/10.1007/s00276-021-02757-y.
58. Yazar F, Imre N, Battal B, Bilgic S, Tayfun C. Is there any relation between distal parameters of the femur and its height and width? Surg Radiol Anat. 2011; https://doi.org/10.1007/s00276-011-0847-1.
59. Murshed KA, Çiçekcibaşi AE, Karabacakoğlu A, Şeker M, Ziylan T. Distal femur morphometry: a gender and bilateral comparative study using magnetic resonance imaging. Surg Radiol Anat. 2004; https://doi.org/10.1007/s00276-004-0295-2.
60. Bozkurt M, Unlu S, Cay N, Apaydin N, Dogan M. The potential effect of anatomic relationship between the femur and the tibia on medial meniscus tears. Surg Radiol Anat. 2014; https://doi.org/10.1007/s00276-014-1266-x.
61. Imre N, Battal B, Acikel CH, Akgun V, Comert A, Yazar F. The demonstration of the number, course, and the location of nutrient artery canals of the femur by multidetector computed tomography. Surg Radiol Anat. 2012; https://doi.org/10.1007/s00276-011-0930-7.

Chapter 6
The Tibial Anatomy

Alfred J. Tria Jr. and Giles R. Scuderi

Machine Generated Summaries

Disclaimer: The summaries in this chapter were generated from Springer Nature publications using abstractive AI auto-summarization: An abstraction-based summarizer creates new text based on deep learning. New phrases are created to summarize the content. As the constituted sentences are machine selected, they may not fully reflect the body of the work, so we strongly advise that the original content is read and cited. The auto-generated summaries were curated by the editor to meet Springer Nature publication standards.

Machine generated keywords: pt, tibial, pco, turkish, pco pt, gerdys, gerdys tubercle, vivo, tubercle, mediolateral dimension, matrix, plate, plate model, model, chinese

Measurement of Femoral Posterior Condylar Offset and Posterior Tibial Slope in Normal Knees Based on 3D Reconstruction [45]

This is a machine-generated summary of:

Bao, Liangxiao; Rong, Shengwei; Shi, Zhanjun; Wang, Jian; Zhang, Yang: Measurement of femoral posterior condylar offset and posterior tibial slope in normal knees based on 3D reconstruction [45]

A. J. Tria Jr. (✉)
Department of Orthopedics, Rutgers-Robert Wood Johnson Medical School, New Brunswick, NJ, USA

G. R. Scuderi
Northwell Health Orthopaedic Institute, New York, NY, USA

A. J. Tria Jr., G. R. Scuderi (eds.), *Ligaments of the Knee*,
https://doi.org/10.1007/978-3-031-66615-5_6

Published in: BMC Musculoskeletal Disorders (2021)
Link to original: https://doi.org/10.1186/s12891-021-04367-6

If you want to cite the papers, please refer to the original.

For technical reasons we could not place the page where the original quote is coming from.

Research Highlights

Total knee arthroplasty (TKA) is a widely performed surgical procedure to alleviate pain and restore function in patients with severe knee joint disorders, such as osteoarthritis. Precise reconstruction of the knee's anatomical alignment is crucial for optimal postoperative outcomes, with the posterior condylar offset (PCO) and the posterior tibial slope (PTS) being key variables influencing range of motion (ROM). Despite their importance, there is a lack of normative data on PCO and PTS in non-pathological knees, which is essential for improving TKA techniques and prosthetic designs. Bao et al. investigated the variability of PCO and PTS in healthy individuals using multi-slice CT scans.

Bao recruited 80 healthy volunteers who underwent CT scans from which PCO and PTS were measured using established protocols. The researchers ensured high reliability in their measurements, as evidenced by satisfactory intraclass correlation coefficients. Their analysis revealed normal distribution patterns for both PCO and PTS across medial and lateral compartments, with notable differences between genders. The study found that males typically had larger PCO but smaller medial PTS compared to females. Furthermore, an inverse correlation between PCO and PTS was observed in the medial compartment, suggesting a complex interplay affecting knee flexion and stability.

The findings provide normative data on PCO and PTS, and highlight the importance of considering individual anatomical variations, including gender differences, when planning TKA. The inverse correlation between medial PCO and PTS could have implications for achieving sagittal balance during knee flexion, potentially informing future prosthetic designs that accommodate these variations. As TKA continues to evolve, incorporating such detailed anatomical insights will be crucial for enhancing surgical precision and patient outcomes. Moving forward, research may focus on how these normative values can be applied across diverse populations and age groups to further refine TKA techniques and prosthetic functionality.

Radiographic Measurement of the Posterior Tibial Slope in Normal Chinese Adults: A Retrospective Cohort Study [46]

This is a machine-generated summary of:

Chen, Yong; Ding, Jianping; Dai, Siyu; Yang, Jiao; Wang, Mengke; Tian, Tian; Deng, Xiaolong; Li, Boyi; Cheng, Guohua; Liu, Jie: Radiographic measurement of the posterior tibial slope in normal Chinese adults: a retrospective cohort study [46]

Published in: BMC Musculoskeletal Disorders (2022)

Link to original: https://doi.org/10.1186/s12891-022-05319-4

If you want to cite the papers, please refer to the original.

For technical reasons we could not place the page where the original quote is coming from.

Research Highlights

The posterior tibial slope (PTS) is a critical anatomical angle influencing knee joint stability and biomechanics, essential for surgical procedures such as total knee arthroplasty and anterior cruciate ligament reconstruction. Variations in PTS can lead to significant clinical symptoms, including increased risk of ACL injury or aseptic loosening of knee prostheses. Despite its importance, there is a lack of consensus on the average PTS values across different populations, particularly in the Chinese demographic. Chen et al. addresses this knowledge gap by determining the mean PTS in healthy Chinese adults and examining its correlation with sex, age, and side of the knee.

Utilizing the Picture Archiving and Communication System (PACS), Chen retrospectively analyzed knee radiographs from patients at the Affiliated Hospital of Hangzhou Normal University. They selected subjects based on strict inclusion and exclusion criteria to ensure accurate PTS measurements using GE Centricity PACS software and the anterior tibial cortex method. The study included interobserver and intraobserver reliability analyses, revealing high consistency in PTS measurements. Statistical analyses demonstrated significant differences in PTS values between sexes and among various age groups but not between left and right knees.

This comprehensive study marks a significant advance in understanding the PTS in the Chinese population, highlighting notable differences based on sex and age. These findings underscore the necessity for personalized approaches in knee surgeries within this demographic. The data from this study could help provide guidance for knee surgery and prosthesis manufacturers. Looking ahead, they advocate for further research to refine these findings across diverse ethnicities and regions within China, as well as the development of AI-assisted measurement tools to enhance precision in future studies.

Evaluation of the Relationship of Posterior Tibial Slope with Gender and Age in Turkish Population with 3 Different Methods [47]

This is a machine-generated summary of:

Kavak, Seyhmus; Kaya, Sehmuz: Evaluation of the relationship of posterior tibial slope with gender and age in Turkish population with 3 different methods [47]

Published in: BMC Musculoskeletal Disorders (2024)

Link to original: https://doi.org/10.1186/s12891-024-07209-3

If you want to cite the papers, please refer to the original.

For technical reasons we could not place the page where the original quote is coming from.

Research Highlights

The posterior tibial slope (PTS) is a critical anatomical angle influencing knee joint function and stability, with implications for surgical outcomes in procedures such as total knee arthroplasty (TKA) and anterior cruciate ligament (ACL) reconstruction. Despite its importance, variations in PTS measurement methods and patient demographics have led to inconsistent findings across studies. Kavak et al. investigated the mean PTS angles in the Turkish population, examining the influence of gender and age, and evaluating the repeatability of various measurement techniques.

Kavak conducted a retrospective analysis of lateral knee radiographs from patients who visited an emergency department and orthopedic outpatient clinic. Utilizing GXR-SD devices for image acquisition and OsiriX MD software for evaluation, they measured PTS angles using anterior tibial cortex (ATC), proximal tibial anatomical axis (PTAA), and fibular shaft axis methods. The study included independent measurements by a radiologist and an orthopedist, with a blinded radiologist repeating measurements to ensure reliability. Statistical analyses were performed using SPSS software, focusing on mean PTS angles across different methods, gender, age groups, and interobserver correlations.

The study revealed significant age-related differences in PTS angles but found no gender-based differences when accounting for age. The PTAA method showed the highest intraobserver and interobserver agreement, suggesting it as a reliable technique for clinical use. While the study advances our understanding of PTS variations within the Turkish population, Kavak acknowledges limitations such as excluding patients with degenerative arthritis or those over 60 years old. Future research could benefit from multicenter studies to generalize findings across diverse populations and include weight and height data to explore their relationship with PTS angles further.

Ex Vivo Cortical Porosity and Thickness Predictions at the Tibia Using Full-Spectrum Ultrasonic Guided-Wave Analysis [48]

This is a machine-generated summary of:

Schneider, Johannes; Iori, Gianluca; Ramiandrisoa, Donatien; Hammami, Maroua; Gräsel, Melanie; Chappard, Christine; Barkmann, Reinhard; Laugier, Pascal; Grimal, Quentin; Minonzio, Jean-Gabriel; Raum, Kay: Ex vivo cortical porosity and thickness predictions at the tibia using full-spectrum ultrasonic guided-wave analysis [48]

Published in: Archives of Osteoporosis (2019)

Research Highlights

Postmenopausal women experience significant bone loss from the cortical compartment, with reductions in cortical thickness (Ct.Th) and increases in cortical porosity (Ct.Po), both of which are linked to a higher risk of hip fractures. High-resolution peripheral quantitative computed tomography (HR-pQCT) can measure these parameters but is limited by its availability and use of ionizing radiation. Schneider et al. explored the use of axial transmission (AT) ultrasound, a non-ionizing alternative, to predict Ct.Th and Ct.Po in human tibia samples ex vivo, potentially offering a more accessible and safer method for assessing fracture risk.

Schneider employed a model-based inversion method using AT ultrasound to estimate Ct.Th and Ct.Po, comparing these predictions with site-matched reference measurements obtained through micro-computed tomography (μCT). They designed a novel probe optimized for the tibial diaphysis, which allowed for the excitation of guided waves within the cortical bone's thickness range found in humans. The researchers accounted for variations in bone matrix elasticity by incorporating acoustic impedance measurements from scanning acoustic microscopy (SAM), challenging the assumption that matrix stiffness is invariant across specimens.

The study examined 19 left tibia specimens from human cadavers provided by the Institute of Anatomy at the University of Lübeck. Measurements were performed using their custom-made probe and advanced signal processing techniques to extract velocity data from guided waves. Their approach corrected for potential errors such as small inclination angles between the probe and bone surface, ensuring accurate estimations of Ct.Th and Ct.Po.

The main advance reported by Schneider is the successful validation of AT ultrasound against μCT for estimating Ct.Th and Ct.Po in human tibia samples ex vivo. The findings suggest that variations in matrix stiffness have a minor impact on effective elasticity tensor compared to porosity effects. However, they observed an overestimation of Ct.Th by AT in samples with irregular boundaries, indicating that further research is needed to understand wave behavior in such cases fully.

The study points towards future directions where full-spectrum ultrasonic guided-wave analysis could be applied in vivo, offering a promising tool for osteoporosis diagnosis and fracture risk prediction without ionizing radiation. Schneider noted that further studies are currently ongoing to confirm the possibility of a full-spectrum ultrasonic guided-wave analysis in vivo, highlighting the potential for this technology to move from the lab to clinical practice.

Reappraisal of the Proximal Tibia Anatomy in Turkish Population [49]

This is a machine-generated summary of:

Akdemir Aktaş, Hilal; Ülkir, Mehmet; Günenç Beşer, Ceren; Demiryürek, Deniz: Reappraisal of the proximal tibia anatomy in Turkish population [49]

Published in: Surgical and Radiologic Anatomy (2023)

Link to original: https://doi.org/10.1007/s00276-023-03094-y

If you want to cite the papers, please refer to the original.

For technical reasons we could not place the page where the original quote is coming from.

Research Highlights

Total knee arthroplasty (TKA) is a critical surgical procedure increasingly utilized to address late-stage knee osteoarthritis, with the success of the surgery heavily reliant on the precise sizing of the tibial implant. This sizing is contingent upon a thorough understanding of the proximal tibial anatomy, which includes various structures such as the medial and lateral condyles, intercondylar area, and the tibial tuberosity. Despite its importance, there is a paucity of data on the morphometry of these structures in the Turkish population, which could be pivotal for optimizing prosthetic design. Aktaş et al. performed a comprehensive analysis of proximal tibia and Gerdy's tubercle morphometry, aiming to establish guidelines for TKA prostheses tailored to the Turkish population.

The research examined human dry tibiae from Turkish adults, with ethical approval from Hacettepe University's ethics committee. The study measured various dimensions of the tibial plateau and Gerdy's tubercle using calibrated instruments, ensuring high inter-rater reliability. The parameters assessed included anteroposterior and mediolateral measurements of tibial condyles, intercondylar area dimensions, and details regarding Gerdy's tubercle's shape and texture.

Statistical analyses were conducted to determine significant differences and correlations among these measurements.

The findings revealed notable asymmetry between medial and lateral tibial condyles, with medial condyle dimensions being significantly larger—a fact that could have profound implications for prosthetic design. Additionally, the study highlighted the first-time measurement of certain dimensions related to Gerdy's tubercle, offering new insights into this anatomical landmark's variability.

This study. marks an advance in our understanding of proximal tibial anatomy within the Turkish population. It underscores the necessity for patient-specific prosthetic components that accommodate anatomical variations—potentially reducing implant mismatches and improving surgical outcomes. The data obtained from this study can be used as a guideline in designing tibial components of total knee prostheses. Furthermore, recognizing differences in anteroposterior dimensions between medial and lateral tibial condyles could lead to more individualized knee implant designs.

While this research provides valuable morphometric data, it also highlights future research opportunities such as exploring gender- and age-related anatomical differences using advanced imaging techniques. Such studies could further refine prosthetic designs to achieve personalized medicine in TKA.

Bibliography

1. Arabori M, Matsui N, Kuroda R, Mizuno K, Doita M, Kurosaka M, et al. Posterior condylar offset and flexion in posterior cruciate-retaining and posterior stabilized TKA. J Orthop Sci. 2008;13(1):46–50. https://doi.org/10.1007/s00776-007-1191-5.
2. Bellemans J, Banks S, Victor J, Vandenneucker H, Moemans A. Fluoroscopic analysis of the kinematics of deep flexion in total knee arthroplasty. Influence of posterior condylar offset. J Bone Joint Surg Br. 2002;84(1):50–3. https://doi.org/10.1302/0301-620X.84B1.0840050.
3. Malviya A, Lingard EA, Weir DJ, Deehan DJ. Predicting range of movement after knee replacement: the importance of posterior condylar offset and tibial slope. Knee Surg Sports Traumatol Arthrosc. 2009;17(5):491–8. https://doi.org/10.1007/s00167-008-0712-x.
4. Massin P, Gournay A. Optimization of the posterior condylar offset, tibial slope, and condylar roll-back in total knee arthroplasty. J Arthroplast. 2006;21(6):889–96. https://doi.org/10.1016/j.arth.2005.10.019.
5. Zhang Y, Wang J, Xiao J, Zhao L, Li ZH, Yan G, et al. Measurement and comparison of tibial posterior slope angle in different methods based on three-dimensional reconstruction. Knee. 2014;21(3):694–8. https://doi.org/10.1016/j.knee.2014.01.008.
6. Bauer T, Biau D, Colmar M, Poux X, Hardy P, Lortat-Jacob A. Influence of posterior condylar offset on knee flexion after cruciate-sacrificing mobile-bearing total knee replacement: a prospective analysis of 410 consecutive cases. Knee. 2010;17(6):375–80. https://doi.org/10.1016/j.knee.2009.11.001.
7. Cinotti G, Sessa P, Ripani FR, Postacchini R, Masciangelo R, Giannicola G. Correlation between posterior offset of femoral condyles and sagittal slope of the tibial plateau. J Anat. 2012;221(5):452–8. https://doi.org/10.1111/j.1469-7580.2012.01563.x.
8. Hashemi J, Chandrashekar N, Gill B, Beynnon BD, Slauterbeck JR, Schutt RC Jr, et al. The geometry of the tibial plateau and its influence on the biomechanics of the tibiofemoral joint. J Bone Joint Surg Am. 2008;90(12):2724–34. https://doi.org/10.2106/JBJS.G.01358.

9. Kang KT, Koh YG, Son J, Kwon OR, Lee JS, Kwon SK. A computational simulation study to determine the biomechanical influence of posterior condylar offset and tibial slope in cruciate retaining total knee arthroplasty. Bone Joint Res. 2018;7(1):69–78. https://doi.org/10.1302/2046-3758.71.BJR-2017-0143.R1.
10. Laskin RS, Riegèr MA. The surgical technique for performing a total knee replacement arthroplasty. Orthop Clin North Am. 1989;20(1):31–48.
11. Malek IA, Moorehead JD, Abiddin Z, Montgomery SC. The correlation between femoral condyle radii and subject height. Clin Anat. 2009;22(4):517–22. https://doi.org/10.1002/ca.20787.
12. Matsuda S, Miura H, Nagamine R, Urabe K, Ikenoue T, Okazaki K, et al. Posterior tibial slope in the normal and varus knee. Am J Knee Surg. 1999;12(3):165–8.
13. Han HS, Chang CB, Seong SC, Lee S, Lee MC. Evaluation of anatomic references for tibial sagittal alignment in total knee arthroplasty. Knee Surg Sports Traumatol Arthrosc. 2008;16(4):373–7. https://doi.org/10.1007/s00167-008-0486-1.
14. Voleti PB, Stephenson JW, Lotke PA, Lee GC. Plain radiographs underestimate the asymmetry of the posterior condylar offset of the knee compared with MRI. Clin Orthop Relat Res. 2014;472(1):155–61. https://doi.org/10.1007/s11999-013-2946-2.
15. Bernhardson AS, DePhillipo NN, Daney BT, Kennedy MI, Aman ZS, LaPrade RF. Posterior Tibial slope and risk of posterior cruciate ligament injury. Am J Sports Med. 2019;47(2):312–7. https://doi.org/10.1177/0363546518819176.
16. Giffin JR, Vogrin TM, Zantop T, et al. Effects of increasing tibial slope on the biomechanics of the knee. Am J Sports Med. 2004;32(2):376–82. https://doi.org/10.1177/0363546503258880.
17. Khattak MJ, Umer M, Davis ET, Habib M, Ahmed M. Lower-limb alignment and posterior tibial slope in Pakistanis: a radiographic study. J Orthop Surg (Hong Kong). 2010;18(1):22–5. https://doi.org/10.1177/230949901001800105.
18. Webb JM, Salmon LJ, Leclerc E, Pinczewski LA, Roe JP. Posterior tibial slope and further anterior cruciate ligament injuries in the anterior cruciate ligament-reconstructed patient. Am J Sports Med. 2013;41(12):2800–4. https://doi.org/10.1177/0363546513503288.
19. Song GY, Zhang H, Zhang J, Liu X, Xue Z, et al. Greater static anterior tibial subluxation of the lateral compartment after an acute anterior cruciate ligament injury is associated with an increased posterior tibial slope. Am J Sports Med. 2018;46(7):1617–23. https://doi.org/10.1177/0363546518760580.
20. Yoo JH, Chang CB, Shin KS, Seong SC, Kim TK. Anatomical references to assess the posterior tibial slope in total knee arthroplasty: a comparison of 5 anatomical axes. J Arthroplast. 2008;23(4):586–92. https://doi.org/10.1016/j.arth.2007.05.006.
21. Hohmann E, Bryant A, Reaburn P, Tetsworth K. Is there a correlation between posterior tibial slope and non-contact anterior cruciate ligament injuries? Knee Surg Sports Traumatol Arthrosc. 2011;19(Suppl 1):S109–14. https://doi.org/10.1007/s00167-011-1547-4.
22. Chambers AW, Wood AR, Kosmopoulos V, Sanchez HB, Wagner RA. Effect of posterior tibial slope on flexion and anterior-posterior tibial translation in posterior cruciate-retaining total knee arthroplasty. J Arthroplast. 2016;31(1):103–6. https://doi.org/10.1016/j.arth.2015.08.027.
23. Aljuaid MO, El-Ghamry OR. Determination of epiphyseal union age in the knee and hand joints bones among the Saudi population in Taif City. Radiol Res Pract. 2018;2018:7854287. https://doi.org/10.1155/2018/7854287. PMID: 29888003; PMCID:PMC5985073.
24. Washburn SL. Skeletal age changes in young American males, analyzed from the standpoint of age identifcation. Tomas W. McKern and T. D. Stewart. Technical Report EP-45, Environmental Protection Research Division, Quartermaster Research and Development Center, U.S. Army, Natick, 1957. viii+ 179 pp., 87 fgs., 52 tables. Am Antiq. 1958;24(2):198–9.
25. Schaefer MC, Black SM. Comparison of ages of epiphyseal union in north American and Bosnian skeletal material. J Forensic Sci. 2005;50(4):777–84.
26. O'Connor JE, Bogue C, Spence LD, Last J. A method to establish the relationship between chronological age and stage of union from radiographic assessment of epiphyseal fusion at the knee: an Irish population study. J Anat. 2008;212(2):198–209. https://doi.org/10.1111/j.1469-7580.2007.00847.x. Epub 2008 Jan 3.PMID: 18179475; PMCID: PMC2408977.

27. Chiu KY, Zhang SD, Zhang GH. Posterior slope of tibial plateau in Chinese. J Arthroplast. 2000;15(2):224–7. https://doi.org/10.1016/s0883-5403(00)90330-9.
28. Brazier J, Migaud H, Gougeon F, Cotten A, Fontaine C, Duquennoy A. Evaluation des méthodes de mesure radiographique de la pente tibiale. Analyse De 83 genoux témoins [Evaluation of methods for radiographic measurement of the tibial slope. A study of 83 healthy knees]. Rev Chir Orthop Reparatrice Appar Mot. 1996;82:195–200.
29. Hernigou P, Goutallier D. Usure osseuse sous-chondrale des plateaux tibiaux dans les gonarthroses fémoro-tibiales. Aspect radiologique sur l'incidence de profil. Corrélations cliniques, anatomiques et conséquences [Subchondral bone wear of the tibial plateau in femorotibial knee osteoarthritis. Radiologic aspects in the profile incidence. Clinical, anatomical correlations and consequences]. Rev Rhum Mal Osteoartic. 1990;57:67–72.
30. Ho WP, Cheng CK, Liau JJ. Morphometrical measurements of resected surface of femurs in Chinese knees: correlation to the sizing of current femoral implants. Knee. 2006;13:12–4.
31. Julliard R, Genin P, Weil G, Palmkrantz P. La Pente tibiale fonctionnelle médiane. Principe. Technique de mesure. Valeur. Intérêt [The median functional slope of the tibia. Principle. Technique of measurement. Value Interest]. Rev Chir Orthop Reparatrice Appar Mot. 1993;79:625–34.
32. Chen Y, Ding J, Dai S, Yang J, Wang M, Tian T, et al. Radiographic measurement of the posterior tibial slope in normal Chinese adults: a retrospective cohort study. BMC Musculoskelet Disord. 2022;23:386.
33. Medda S, Kundu R, Sengupta S, Pal AK. Anatomical variation of posterior slope of tibial plateau in adult eastern Indian population. Indian J Orthop. 2017;51(1):69–74. https://doi.org/10.4103/0019-5413.197545.
34. Karjalainen J, Riekkinen O, Töyräs J, et al. Ultrasonic assessment of cortical bone thickness in vitro and in vivo. IEEE Trans Ultrason Ferroelectr Freq Control. 2008;55:2191–7. https://doi.org/10.1109/TUFFC.918.
35. Minonzio J-G, Talmant M, Laugier P. Guided wave phase velocity measurement using multi-emitter and multi-receiver arrays in the axial transmission configuration. J Acoust Soc Am. 2010;127:2913–9. https://doi.org/10.1121/1.3377085.
36. Talmant M, Kolta S, Roux C, Haguenauer D, Vedel I, Cassou B, Bossy E, Laugier P. In vivo performance evaluation of bi-directional ultrasonic axial transmission for cortical bone assessment. Ultrasound Med Biol. 2009;35:912–9. https://doi.org/10.1016/j.ultrasmedbio.2008.12.008.
37. Moilanen P, Määttä M, Kilappa V, Xu L, Nicholson PHF, Alén M, Timonen J, Jämsä T, Cheng S. Discrimination of fractures by low-frequency axial transmission ultrasound in postmenopausal females. Osteoporos Int. 2012;24:723–30. https://doi.org/10.1007/s00198-012-2022-x.
38. Knapp KM, Blake GM, Fogelman I, et al. Multisite quantitative ultrasound: Colles' fracture discrimination in postmenopausal women. Osteoporos Int J Establ Result Coop Eur Found Osteoporos Natl Osteoporos Found USA. 2002;13:474–9. https://doi.org/10.1007/s001980200057.
39. Bossy E, Talmant M, Laugier P. Bi-directional axial transmission improves accuracy and precision of ultrasonic velocity measurement in cortical bone. IEEE Trans Ultrason Ferroelectr Freq Control. 2004;51(1):71–9.
40. Moilanen P, Nicholson PHF, Kilappa V, Cheng S, Timonen J. Assessment of the cortical bone thickness using ultrasonic guided waves: modelling and in vitro study. Ultrasound Med Biol. 2007;33:254–62. https://doi.org/10.1016/j.ultrasmedbio.2006.07.038.
41. Tatarinov A, Sarvazyan A, Beller G, Felsenberg D. Comparative examination of human proximal tibiae in vitro by ultrasonic guided waves and pQCT. Ultrasound Med Biol. 2011;37:1791–801. https://doi.org/10.1016/j.ultrasmedbio.2011.04.013.
42. Kwak DS, Surendran S, Pengatteeri YH, Park SE, Choi KN, Gopinathan P, et al. Morphometry of the proximal tibia to design the tibial component of total knee arthroplasty for the Korean population. Knee. 2007;14:295–300.

43. Dai Y, Bischoff JE. Comprehensive assessment of tibial plateau morphology in total knee arthroplasty: Influence of shape and size on anthropometric variability. J Orthop Res. 2013;31(10):1643–52. https://doi.org/10.1002/jor.22410.
44. Gandhi S, Singla RK, Kullar JS, Suri RK, Mehta V. Morphometric analysis of upper end of tibia. J Clin Diagn Res. 2014;8(8):10–3. https://doi.org/10.7860/jcdr/2014/8973.4736.
45. Bao L, Rong S, Shi Z, Wang J, Zhang Y. Measurement of femoral posterior condylar offset and posterior tibial slope in normal knees based on 3D reconstruction. BMC Musculoskelet Disord. 2021;22(1):486. https://doi.org/10.1186/s12891-021-04367-6.
46. Chen Y, Ding J, Dai S, Yang J, Wang M, Tian T, Deng X, Li B, Cheng G, Liu J. Radiographic measurement of the posterior tibial slope in normal Chinese adults: a retrospective cohort study. BMC Musculoskelet Disord. 2022;23(1):386. https://doi.org/10.1186/s12891-022-05319-4.
47. Kavak S, Kaya S. Evaluation of the relationship of posterior tibial slope with gender and age in Turkish population with 3 different methods. BMC Musculoskelet Disord. 2024;25(1):102. https://doi.org/10.1186/s12891-024-07209-3.
48. Schneider J, Iori G, Ramiandrisoa D, Hammami M, Gräsel M, Chappard C, Barkmann R, Laugier P, Grimal Q, Minonzio J-G, Raum K. Ex vivo cortical porosity and thickness predictions at the tibia using full-spectrum ultrasonic guided-wave analysis. Arch Osteoporos. 2019;14(1):21. https://doi.org/10.1007/s11657-019-0578-1.
49. Akdemir Aktaş H, Ülkir M, Günenç Beşer C, Demiryürek D. Reappraisal of the proximal tibia anatomy in Turkish population. Surg Radiol Anat. 2023;45(3):263–70. https://doi.org/10.1007/s00276-023-03094-y.

Chapter 7
The Patellar Anatomy

Alfred J. Tria Jr. and Giles R. Scuderi

Machine Generated Summaries

Disclaimer: The summaries in this chapter were generated from Springer Nature publications using abstractive AI auto-summarization: An abstraction-based summarizer creates new text based on deep learning. New phrases are created to summarize the content. As the constituted sentences are machine selected, they may not fully reflect the body of the work, so we strongly advise that the original content is read and cited. The auto-generated summaries were curated by the editor to meet Springer Nature publication standards.

Machine generated keywords: patellar, patella, patellofemoral, patella patellar, patellar tendon, tendon, mpfc, method, patellar ligament, cubiti, patella cubiti, ratio, medial patellofemoral, fiber, use distal

The Geometry of Patella and Patellar Tendon Measured on Knee MRI [26]

This is a machine-generated summary of:

Yoo, Jae Ho; Yi, Seung Rim; Kim, Jin Hong: The geometry of patella and patellar tendon measured on Knee MRI [26]

Published in: Surgical and Radiologic Anatomy (2007)

Link to original: https://doi.org/10.1007/s00276-007-0261-x

A. J. Tria Jr. (✉)
Department of Orthopedics, Rutgers-Robert Wood Johnson Medical School, New Brunswick, NJ, USA

G. R. Scuderi
Northwell Health Orthopaedic Institute, New York, NY, USA

A. J. Tria Jr., G. R. Scuderi (eds.), *Ligaments of the Knee*, https://doi.org/10.1007/978-3-031-66615-5_7

If you want to cite the papers, please refer to the original.

For technical reasons we could not place the page where the original quote is coming from.

Research Highlights

The patella, as the largest sesamoid bone, plays a crucial role in enhancing the quadriceps muscle's extension capacity by acting as a biomechanical lever arm. Despite its clinical importance, there remains a significant knowledge gap in quantitative anatomical data regarding the patella and patellar tendon—data that are essential for understanding knee mechanics and pathologies, as well as for informing surgical practices such as anterior cruciate ligament reconstruction and total knee arthroplasty. Yoo et al., using MRI measurements provides a comprehensive analysis on the morphology of the patella and patellar tendon.

Yoo measured 172 knees from subjects with specific inclusion and exclusion criteria to ensure the reliability of their findings. The team measured specific dimensions of the patella and patellar tendon using multi-slice, weighted non-fat-saturated conventional spin-echo images. They standardized their imaging protocol to minimize discrepancies between actual structures and their representations in MRI images. Their measurements were conducted with precision to ensure reliability.

The study found significant differences in the geometry of these structures between male and female subjects, with men generally having larger patellae and tendons. Moreover, while the overall geometry of the patella correlated well with anthropometric measures such as weight, height, and BMI, this was not the case for the patellar tendon. The authors highlight that the thickness of the patella showed a strong correlation with anthropometric measures, which is crucial for surgical procedures aiming to restore normal knee mechanics.

This study provides normative data on the geometry of the patella and patellar tendon. These findings have important implications for surgical practices, particularly in reconstructive procedures where accurate restoration of anatomy is critical for optimal outcomes. This research should serve as a foundation for future research.

Future Directions in Patellofemoral Imaging and 3D Modeling [49]

This is a machine-generated summary of:

Dandu, Navya; Knapik, Derrick M.; Trasolini, Nicholas A.; Zavras, Athan G.; Yanke, Adam B.: Future Directions in Patellofemoral Imaging and 3D Modeling [49]

Published in: Current Reviews in Musculoskeletal Medicine (2022)
Link to original: https://doi.org/10.1007/s12178-022-09746-7

If you want to cite the papers, please refer to the original.

For technical reasons we could not place the page where the original quote is coming from.

Research Highlights

The patellofemoral joint's function is a complex interplay of static and dynamic restraints, with accurate diagnosis and surgical planning hinging on understanding the pathoanatomy involved in maltracking or instability. Traditional imaging techniques like radiographs and MRI scans have limitations, such as operator dependency and inability to assess cartilaginous surfaces accurately. Dandu et al. addresses these challenges by exploring evolving techniques in patellofemoral imaging, including dynamic assessments, automation of measurement, and advanced predictive computer modeling.

Dandu delves into the intricacies of patellofemoral joint evaluation, underscoring the inadequacy of two-dimensional imaging for capturing the three-dimensional nature of patellar maltracking. The study employs a variety of advanced imaging modalities, including three-dimensional MRI reconstructions and dynamic imaging techniques like weightbearing MRI and CT scans. Their findings highlight the dynamic changes in patellar tracking that cannot be appreciated with static imaging.. By integrating automated detection software with customized algorithms, the team has significantly reduced inter-rater variability, paving the way for more reliable and comprehensive diagnostic tools.

The study also emphasizes the importance of dynamic assessment in clinical settings. The authors found that upright weightbearing conditions significantly affect measurements such as patellar height and tilt angle, which are crucial for surgical decision-making. Dynamic conditions provide a more accurate representation of the patient's anatomy during activity.. The research further explores the potential of machine learning to automate measurement processes, thereby normalizing values for better treatment guidance.

The advancements presented by Dandu et al. mark significant progress in patellofemoral joint imaging. The shift from static to dynamic assessment techniques offers a more accurate depiction of patellar tracking and its contributing factors. Their work sets the stage for future developments in three-dimensional classification systems and predictive modeling, pointing towards a horizon where automated measurements and finite element analysis models could revolutionize preoperative planning and postoperative assessment. While these innovative approaches show promise, they require clinical validation and integration into routine practice to truly transform patient care in orthopedics.

Novel Method of Measuring Patellar Height Ratio Using a Distal Femoral Reference Point [50]

This is a machine-generated summary of:

Chareancholvanich, Keerati; Narkbunnam, Rapeepat: Novel method of measuring patellar height ratio using a distal femoral reference point [50]

Published in: International Orthopaedics (2011)

Link to original: https://doi.org/10.1007/s00264-011-1340-5

If you want to cite the papers, please refer to the original.

For technical reasons we could not place the page where the original quote is coming from.

Research Highlights

The patellofemoral joint is crucial for knee extension, with patellar height playing a significant role in joint mechanics and associated conditions such as patellofemoral pain and instability. Despite various measurement methods, there is no consensus on the best approach, particularly one that remains accurate across different knee flexion angles. Now a new study Chareancholvanich et al. introduces a novel method for measuring patellar height using the distal femur as a reference point, aiming to provide consistent results irrespective of knee flexion angle.

In this study, 85 volunteers underwent lateral radiographs at multiple angles of knee flexion to assess the accuracy and reproducibility of the new measurement method compared to existing ones. The researchers used a custom adjustable frame and goniometric ruler to standardize knee positioning, ensuring high-quality radiographic control. The new method calculates the ratio between the distance from the posterior angle of the intercondylar roof to the tibial tubercle and the midpoint of the patellar articular facet to the tibial tubercle. Statistical analysis demonstrated that this novel method yielded consistent normal values across different degrees of knee flexion, unlike some traditional methods which varied significantly with flexion angle.

Chareancholvanich introduces a new advance in patellar height measurement by developing a method that maintains accuracy across varying degrees of knee flexion, with high interobserver reliability. The study's findings suggest that this new approach could become a valuable clinical tool for diagnosing and treating knee conditions. Their proposed novel patellar height-ratio measurement index is an accurate and promising method for evaluating patellar height in the normal population. This research paves the way for future studies to validate this method in pathological knees and potentially establish it as a new standard for clinical practice.

Morphometric Analysis of Patella and Patellar Ligament: A Cadaveric Study to Aid Patellar Tendon Grafts [51]

This is a machine-generated summary of:

Aithal Padur, Ashwini; Kumar, Naveen; Lewis, Melissa Glenda; Sekaran, Varalakshmi Chandra: Morphometric analysis of patella and patellar ligament: a cadaveric study to aid patellar tendon grafts [51]

Published in: Surgical and Radiologic Anatomy (2021)

Link to original: https://doi.org/10.1007/s00276-021-02837-z

If you want to cite the papers, please refer to the original.

For technical reasons we could not place the page where the original quote is coming from.

Research Highlights

Anterior cruciate ligament (ACL) injuries are prevalent among athletes, often necessitating surgical intervention using grafts from the patellar ligament or quadriceps tendon to restore knee stability. The patella, integral to the knee extensor mechanism, lacks morphological sex determination and remains structurally resilient postmortem. Despite its clinical importance, there is a paucity of detailed morphometric data on the patella and patellar ligament, particularly for the Indian population, which is critical for accurate diagnoses and surgical interventions. Padur et al. performed comprehensive morphometric measurements of the patellar ligament and its localization through gross anatomical dissections of adult cadavers from the South Indian population.

Padur embarked on an exploration of the anatomy of the patellar ligament, employing formalin-fixed male cadavers to ensure precise measurements devoid of approximation. The researchers dissected the knee region to reveal the quadriceps tendon, patella, and patellar ligament, taking care to preserve their natural state. Measurements were conducted in situ using calibrated tools, with each parameter measured twice to eliminate interobserver variability. The statistical analysis included mean, standard deviation, and median scores for various parameters, with no significant side differences observed between right and left limbs. Spearman's correlation tests further elucidated relationships between different aspects of the patellar anatomy.

This study marks an advance in our understanding of knee morphology, offering insights into the dimensions of the patella and patellar ligament within the South Indian demographic. These findings serve as a reference for designing prosthetic implants tailored to this population. These findings may serve as a foundation for future clinical applications, including improved ACL reconstruction techniques using patellar ligament grafts. While acknowledging limitations such as the use of embalmed cadavers and lack of female specimens, this work paves the way for integrating cadaveric and radiological methods to enhance surgical precision and patient outcomes in orthopedics.

The Medial Patellofemoral Complex [52]

This is a machine-generated summary of:

Loeb, Alexander E.; Tanaka, Miho J.: The medial patellofemoral complex [52]

Published in: Current Reviews in Musculoskeletal Medicine (2018)

Link to original: https://doi.org/10.1007/s12178-018-9475-2

If you want to cite the papers, please refer to the original.

For technical reasons we could not place the page where the original quote is coming from.

Research Highlights

Patellar instability is a prevalent issue among adolescents and young adults, leading to significant knee dysfunction. Despite advancements in treatment, the complexity of the medial patellofemoral complex (MPFC) and its role in patellar stability remains a challenge. Loeb et al. delved into the intricacies of MPFC anatomy, function, and surgical reconstruction, offering insights into improving patient outcomes for those suffering from patellar instability.

Loeb reviewed the evolution of MPFC's anatomical and biomechanical definitions, emphasizing its significance as a restraint against lateral patellar translation. The study employs a combination of methods including cadaveric dissections, radiographic analysis, and computational modeling to elucidate the MPFC's structure and function. The authors highlight the importance of accurate graft placement during reconstruction to replicate the native MPFC's biomechanics. They also explore various surgical techniques, fixation methods, and graft types to determine their effectiveness in restoring patellar stability while minimizing complications.

The research underscores significant advances in MPFC reconstruction, particularly the shift towards techniques that incorporate quadriceps tendon fixation to better mimic natural anatomy. The findings suggest that addressing concomitant pathologies such as tibial tuberosity lateralization, patella alta, and trochlear dysplasia is crucial for successful outcomes. The study also points towards future research directions, including refining surgical techniques to optimize graft function and minimize joint overconstraint. MPFC reconstruction has shown promising results with proper indications; however, continued efforts are needed to standardize procedures and minimize technical errors. This work helps to improve the management of patellar instability through the understanding of MPFC's role in knee biomechanics and targeted surgical interventions.

Bibliography

1. Aglietti P, Insall JN, Walker PS, et al. A new patella prosthesis. Design and application. Clin Orthop. 1975;107:175–87.
2. Baldwin JL, House CK. Anatomic dimensions of the patella measured during total knee arthroplasty. J Arthroplast. 2005;20:250–7.
3. Hofmann AA, Tkach TK, Evanich CJ, et al. Patellar component medialization in total knee arthroplasty. J Arthroplast. 1997;12:155–60.
4. Koh JS, Yeo SJ, Lee BP, et al. Influence of patellar thickness on results of total knee arthroplasty: does a residual bony patellar thickness of ≤12 mm lead to poorer clinical outcome and increased complication rates? J Arthroplast. 2002;17:56–61.
5. Andrikoula S, Tokis A, Vasiliadis HS, et al. The extensor mechanism of the knee joint: an anatomical study. Knee Surg Sports Traumatol Arthrosc. 2006;14:214–20.
6. Dietrich TJ, Fucentese SF, Pfirrmann CW. Imaging of individual anatomical risk factors for patellar instability. In: Seminars in musculoskeletal radiology. Thieme Medical Publishers; 2016. p. 065–73.
7. Aarvold A, Pope A, Sakthivel VK, Ayer RV. MRI performed on dedicated knee coils is inaccurate for the measurement of tibial tubercle trochlear groove distance. Skeletal Radiol. 2014;43(3):345–9. https://doi.org/10.1007/s00256-013-1790-5.
8. Frings J, Dust T, Krause M, Ohlmeier M, Frosch K-H, Adam G, et al. Objective assessment of patellar maltracking with 3 T dynamic magnetic resonance imaging: feasibility of a robust and reliable measuring technique. Sci Rep. 2020;10(1):16770. https://doi.org/10.1038/s41598-020-72332-9. Demonstrated reliability of dynamic MRI technique for evaluation of patellar maltracking and correlation with traditional anatomic factors (e.g. tibial tubercle-trochlear groove (TT-TG) distance, patellar height).
9. Williams AA, Elias JJ, Tanaka MJ, Thawait GK, Demehri S, Carrino JA, Cosgarea AJ. The relationship between tibial tuberosity–trochlear groove distance and abnormal patellar tracking in patients with unilateral patellar instability. Arthrosc J Arthrosc Relat Surg. 2016;32(1):55–61. https://doi.org/10.1016/j.arthro.2015.06.037.
10. Weber AE, Nathani A, Dines JS, Allen AA, Shubin-Stein BE, Arendt EA, Bedi A. An algorithmic approach to the management of recurrent lateral patellar dislocation. J Bone Joint Surg Am. 2016;98(5):417–27. https://doi.org/10.2106/jbjs.O.00354.
11. Suomalainen J-S, Regalado G, Joukainen A, Kääriäinen T, Könönen M, Manninen H, et al. Effects of knee flexion and extension on the tibial tuberosity–trochlear groove (TT–TG) distance in adolescents. J Exp Orthop. 2018;5(1):31. https://doi.org/10.1186/s40634-018-0149-1.

12. Marquez-Lara A, Andersen J, Lenchik L, Ferguson CM, Gupta P. Variability in patellofemoral alignment measurements on MRI: influence of knee position. Am J Roentgenol. 2017;208(5):1097–102. https://doi.org/10.2214/ajr.16.17007.
13. Worden A, Kaar S, Owen J, Cutuk A. Radiographic and anatomic evaluation of tibial tubercle to trochlear groove distance. J Knee Surg. 2016;29(7):589–93. https://doi.org/10.1055/s-0035-1569478.
14. Lenchik L, Heacock L, Weaver AA, Boutin RD, Cook TS, Itri J, Filippi CG, Gullapalli RP, Lee J, Zagurovskaya M, Retson T, Godwin K, Nicholson J, Narayana PA. Automated segmentation of tissues using CT and MRI: a systematic review. Acad Radiol. 2019;26(12):1695–706. https://doi.org/10.1016/j.acra.2019.07.006.
15. Lecun Y, Bengio Y, Hinton G. Deep learning. Nature. 2015;521(7553):436–44. https://doi.org/10.1038/nature14539.
16. Lundervold AS, Lundervold A. An overview of deep learning in medical imaging focusing on MRI. Z Med Phys. 2019;29(2):102–27. https://doi.org/10.1016/j.zemedi.2018.11.002.
17. Litjens G, Kooi T, Bejnordi BE, Setio AAA, Ciompi F, Ghafoorian M, van der Laak JAWM, van Ginneken B, Sánchez CI. A survey on deep learning in medical image analysis. Med Image Anal. 2017;42:60–88. https://doi.org/10.1016/j.media.2017.07.005.
18. Ali AA, Shalhoub SS, Cyr AJ, Fitzpatrick CK, Maletsky LP, Rullkoetter PJ, Shelburne KB. Validation of predicted patellofemoral mechanics in a finite element model of the healthy and cruciate-deficient knee. J Biomech. 2016;49(2):302–9. https://doi.org/10.1016/j.jbiomech.2015.12.020.
19. Kaiser D, Trummler L, Götschi T, Waibel FWA, Snedeker JG, Fucentese SF. Patellofemoral instability in trochleodysplastic knee joints and the quantitative influence of simulated trochleoplasty—a finite element simulation. Clin Biomech (Bristol). 2021;81:105216. https://doi.org/10.1016/j.clinbiomech.2020.105216. Demonstrated feasibility of surgical simulation (trochleoplasty) for a patellofemoral finite element analysis model.
20. Seyahi A, Atalar AC, Koyuncu O, Cinar BM, Demirhan M. Blumensaat line and patellar height. Acta orthop Traumtol Turc. 2006;40(3):240–7.
21. Blumensaat C. Die Lageabweichungen und Verrenkungen der Kniescheibe. Ergebn Chir Orthop. 1938;31:149–223. (in German)
22. Bernageau J, Goutallier D, Debeyre J, Ferrané J. New exploration technic of the patellofemoral joint: relaxed axial quadriceps and contracted quadriceps. Rev Chir Orthop Reparatrice Appar Mot. 1975;61(Suppl 2):286–90. (in French)
23. Biedert RM, Albrecht S. The patellotrochlear index: a new index for assessing patellar height. Knee Surg Sports Traumatol Arthrosc. 2006;14:707–12.
24. Grelsamer RP, Weinstein CH. Applied biomechanics of the patella. Clin Orthop Relat Res. 2001;389:9–14.
25. Miller TT, Staron RB, Feldman F. Patellar height on sagittal MR imaging of the knee. AJR Am J Roentgenol. 1996;167:339–41.
26. Yoo JH, Yi SR, Kim JH. The geometry of patella and patellar tendon measured on knee MRI. Surg Radiol Anat. 2007;29(8):623–8.
27. Schlenzka D, Schwesinger G. The height of the patella: an anatomical study. Eur J Radiol. 1990;11:19–21.
28. Philips CL, Silver DAT, Schranz PJ, Mandalia V. The measurement of patellar height: a review of the methods of imaging. J Bone Jt Surg Br. 2010;92B:1045–53.
29. Portner O, Pakzad H. The evaluation of patellar height: a simple method. J Bone Jt Surg Am. 2011;93:73–80.
30. Potage D, Duparc F, D'Utruy A, Courage O, Roussignol X. Mapping the quadriceps tendon: an anatomic and morphometric study to guide tendon harvesting. Surg Radiol Anat. 2015;37(9):1063–7.
31. Aframian A, Smith TO, Tennent TD, Cobb JP, Hing CB. Origin and insertion of the medial patellofemoral ligament: a systematic review of anatomy. Knee Surg Sport Traumatol Arthrosc. 2016;25:1–18. https://doi.org/10.1007/s00167-016-4272-1.

32. Tanaka MJ. Variability in the patellar attachment of the medial patellofemoral ligament. Arthrosc J Arthrosc Relat Surg. 2016;32(8):1667–70. https://doi.org/10.1016/j.arthro.2016.01.046.
33. Greenrod W, Cox J, Astori I, Baulch J, Williams J. A magnetic resonance imaging study of the significance of the distal femoral physis during medial patellofemoral ligament reconstruction. Orthop J Sport Med. 2013;1(4):232596711350263. https://doi.org/10.1177/2325967113502638.
34. Shea KG, Martinson WD, Cannamela PC, Richmond CG, Fabricant PD, Anderson AF, et al. Variation in the medial patellofemoral ligament origin in the skeletally immature knee: an anatomic study. Am J Sports Med. 2017;46:1–7. https://doi.org/10.1177/0363546517738002.
35. McCulloch PC, Bott A, Ramkumar PN, Suarez A, Isamaily S, Daylamani D, et al. Strain within the native and reconstructed MPFL during knee flexion. J Knee Surg. 2014;27(2):125–31. https://doi.org/10.1055/s-0033-1357496.
36. Wang Q, Huang W, Cai D, Huang H. Biomechanical comparison of single- and double-bundle medial patellofemoral ligament reconstruction. J Orthop Surg Res. 2017;12(1):29. https://doi.org/10.1186/s13018-017-0530-2.
37. Redler L, Meyers K, Munch J, Dennis E, Nguyen J, Stein BS. Anisometry of medial patellofemoral ligament reconstruction in the setting of Patella Alta and increased Tibial tubercle-trochlear groove (TT-TG) distance. Arthrosc J Arthrosc Relat Surg. 2016;32(6):e10. https://doi.org/10.1016/j.arthro.2016.03.054.
38. Stephen JM, Dodds AL, Lumpaopong P, Kader D, Williams A, Amis AA. The ability of medial patellofemoral ligament reconstruction to correct patellar kinematics and contact mechanics in the presence of a lateralized tibial tubercle. Am J Sports Med. 2015;43(9):2198–207. https://doi.org/10.1177/0363546515597906.
39. D'Amore T, Tanaka MJ, Cosgarea AJ. When and how far to move the tibial tuberosity in patients with patellar instability. Sports Med Arthrosc. 2017;25(2):78–84. https://doi.org/10.1097/JSA.0000000000000146.
40. Allen BJ, Krych AJ, Engasser W, Levy BA, Stuart MJ, Collins MS, et al. Medial patellofemoral ligament tears in the setting of multiligament knee injuries rarely cause patellar instability. Am J Sports Med. 2015;43(6):1386–90. https://doi.org/10.1177/0363546515576902.
41. Stephen JM, Kaider D, Lumpaopong P, Deehan DJ, Amis AA. The effect of femoral tunnel position and graft tension on patellar contact mechanics and kinematics after medial patellofemoral ligament reconstruction. Am J Sports Med. 2014;42(2):364–72. https://doi.org/10.1177/0363546513509230.
42. Fulkerson JP, Edgar C. Medial quadriceps tendon-femoral ligament: surgical anatomy and reconstruction technique to prevent patella instability. Arthrosc Tech. 2013;2(2):e125–8. https://doi.org/10.1016/j.eats.2013.01.002. Describes the anatomy of the MQTFL as well as a reconstruction technique that avoids patellar drilling, instead attaching the graft to the deep distal quadriceps tendon.
43. Wang CH, Ma LF, Zhou JW, Ji G, Wang HY, Wang F, et al. Double-bundle anatomical versus single-bundle isometric medial patellofemoral ligament reconstruction for patellar dislocation. Int Orthop. 2013;37(4):617–24. https://doi.org/10.1007/s00264-013-1788-6.
44. Shah JN, Howard JS, Flanigan DC, Brophy RH, Carey JL, Lattermann C. A systematic review of complications and failures associated with medial patellofemoral ligament reconstruction for recurrent patellar dislocation. Am J Sports Med. 2012;40(8):1916–23. https://doi.org/10.1177/0363546512442330.
45. Steiner TM, Torga-Spak R, Teitge RA. Medial patellofemoral ligament reconstruction in patients with lateral patellar instability and trochlear dysplasia. Am J Sports Med. 2006;34(8):1254–61. https://doi.org/10.1177/0363546505285584.
46. Hiemstra LA, Kerslake S, Loewen M, Lafave M. Effect of trochlear dysplasia on outcomes after isolated soft tissue stabilization for patellar instability. Am J Sports Med. 2016;44(6):1515–23. https://doi.org/10.1177/0363546516635626.

47. Hopper GP, Leach WJ, Rooney BP, Walker CR, Blyth MJ. Does degree of trochlear dysplasia and position of femoral tunnel influence outcome after medial patellofemoral ligament reconstruction? Am J Sports Med. 2014;42(3):716–22. https://doi.org/10.1177/0363546513518413.
48. Damasena I, Blythe M, Wysocki D, Kelly D, Annear P. Medial patellofemoral ligament reconstruction combined with distal realignment for recurrent dislocations of the patella: 5-year results of a randomized controlled trial. Am J Sports Med. 2017;45(2):369–76. https://doi.org/10.1177/0363546516666352.
49. Dandu N, Knapik DM, Trasolini NA, Zavras AG, Yanke AB. Future directions in patellofemoral imaging and 3D modeling. Curr Rev Musculoskelet Med. 2022;15(2):82–9. https://doi.org/10.1007/s12178-022-09746-7.
50. Chareancholvanich K, Narkbunnam R. Novel method of measuring patellar height ratio using a distal femoral reference point. Int Orthop. 2011;36(4):749–53. https://doi.org/10.1007/s00264-011-1340-5.
51. Aithal Padur A, Kumar N, Lewis MG, Sekaran VC. Morphometric analysis of patella and patellar ligament: a cadaveric study to aid patellar tendon grafts. Surg Radiol Anat. 2021;43(12):2039–46. https://doi.org/10.1007/s00276-021-02837-z.
52. Loeb AE, Tanaka MJ. The medial patellofemoral complex. Curr Rev Musculoskelet Med. 2018;11(2):201–8. https://doi.org/10.1007/s12178-018-9475-2.

Part III
Kinematics

1.1 Introduction by the Editor

The motion of the knee joint is a combination of flexion/extension, rotation, and anteroposterior motion. The motion is difficult to thoroughly document compromising diagnosis and treatment protocols. As the knee moves from full extension to flexion, the tibia rotates internally because of the greater sagittal motion of the lateral tibiofemoral joint to the medial. The medial tibiofemoral articulation has been likened to a ball-in-socket-joint with minimal motion in the sagittal plane compared to the lateral. The motion of the knee is also dependent upon the forces that are exerted across the joint during the time of the evaluation. Thus, non-weight bearing and full weight bearing studies may vary in their findings. As the knee ages, the ligaments are subject to degenerative changes as are the surfaces of the knee. This leads to changes in mobility and range of motion (ROM). Surgical interventions must consider these changes and whether it is best to try to return the knee to is original pristine function or to accommodate the changes as they present.

The earliest approaches to measuring ROM and kinematics included the use of a goniometer or skin markings. These items are subject to considerable variability due to the placement variation and the mobility of the skin itself. Investigators have looked for improved accuracy and have turned to positional x-rays, dual fluoroscopic imaging systems, MRI, CT, ultrasound, robotic testing, electromagnetic tracking, and surgical navigation. These techniques require advanced imaging equipment that is both time consuming and expensive to implement on a standard clinical basis.

The primary aim of these investigations is to come upon technology that can improve accuracy but at the same time allow ease of application. In the day of increasing costs and prolonged times for development, it would be ideal if simple x-ray or fluoroscopy could answer these demands. Some of the included references show that rather complex evaluations may be correlated with standard applications to increase accuracy in a more functional manner.

Chapter 8 covers the motion of the knee with seven selected references. Yu's article uses two technologies: dual fluoroscopy and MRI. While it is difficult to apply these in the every day setting, the information does add accuracy to the ROM determinations. Bennett's publication uses a digital camera for the analysis and this could have application in the clinical setting. Zlotnicki uses multiple technologies (robotics, surgical navigation, EM tracking) that may help with physical examination standardization but will not be used for routine exams. Kawashima's work shows that the arthritic knee has unique patterns of rotation that may be important for knee replacement designs, perhaps, even moving to individualized prostheses. Hamai studied patellar kinematics using high resolution radiographs and showed the flexion angles increase with greater flexion. This information may help with diagnosis of patellar tracking abnormalities. The final article by Ageberg studied medial-lateral knee motion in flexion and contributes to better evaluation of this motion to screen for knee injury risk.

The classic articles in the bibliography include Dimitriou (the in vivo TEA), DeFrate (patellar tendon function), and Bull (knee motion measurement).

Chapter 9 reviews testing methods and includes six references. Wang was able to developed a lab based method to analyze motion captured data more efficiently. This should make it easier to review data and apply it to developing prosthetic designs for TKA. Wang investigated a portable motion analysis tool and showed that it compares well with biplanar fluoroscopy. This tool uses markers on the skin and processes the data through an automated program. The use of infrared cameras eliminates x-ray exposure and is easier to set up. Bey's study for patellar tracking is CT based. There is x-ray exposure but the high level of accuracy is confirmed with RSA studies. Ohnishi combined bi-plane fluoroscopy and CT to capture dynamic motion which he shows is not the same as the data from static studies. While this is not directly applicable to the clinical settings, it is very helpful in showing the comparison and indicating where static data may not be as precise. Masum's use of ultrasound allowed precision tracking of the motion without the use of x-ray exposure or inhibition of motion. Sander succeeds in modeling the knee joint by incorporating the ligaments and articular cartilage into the dynamic simulations. The virtual tools may help in creating better simulations for surgery.

The classic articles in the bibliography include Zhang (portable motion analysis system), Hume (marker based and stereo radiography kinematics), LaFortune (three dimensional kinematics), and Komistek (fluoroscopic analysis).

Once again, the articles in this chapter are chosen within the Network of Springer publications. Therefore, they are not all inclusive. The generated information is a start to what can be done in the future. The bibliography is less restricted and that is why the editors have added comments about the "classic" articles included in that section. Understanding the ROM and kinematics of the knee is critical for application of ligament reconstructions and knee replacements. It is sometimes difficult to understand the percentage of patients who are disappointed with their surgical result. This is obviously multifactorial. But, it would seem logical to try to replicate the anatomy of the knee with any surgical procedure and the studies in this chapter look towards that solution.

The techniques for measuring the ROM and the associated kinematics are gradually evolving and are improving the level of accuracy. This hopefully will translate into more refined treatment protocols and better clinical results.

Chapter 8
Motion of the Knee

Alfred J. Tria Jr. and Giles R. Scuderi

Machine Generated Summaries

Disclaimer: The summaries in this chapter were generated from Springer Nature publications using abstractive AI auto-summarization: An abstraction-based summarizer creates new text based on deep learning. New phrases are created to summarize the content. As the constituted sentences are machine selected, they may not fully reflect the body of the work, so we strongly advise that the original content is read and cited. The auto-generated summaries were curated by the editor to meet Springer Nature publication standards.

Machine generated keywords: tissue, femoral, response, digital image, digital, patellar, patellar kinematic, loading, load, instability, knee stability, use digital, biomechanical, stability, adaptation

Investigation of Characteristic Motion Patterns of the Knee Joint During a Weightbearing Flexion [25]

This is a machine-generated summary of:

Yu, Jia; Xia, Yulian; Zhou, Chaochao; Tsai, Tsungyuan; Li, Sophia; Foster, Timothy; Bedair, Hany; Li, Guoan: Investigation of Characteristic Motion Patterns of the Knee Joint During a Weightbearing Flexion [25]

Published in: Annals of Biomedical Engineering (2023)

A. J. Tria Jr. (✉)
Department of Orthopedics, Rutgers-Robert Wood Johnson Medical School, New Brunswick, NJ, USA

G. R. Scuderi
Northwell Health Orthopaedic Institute, New York, NY, USA

A. J. Tria Jr., G. R. Scuderi (eds.), *Ligaments of the Knee*,
https://doi.org/10.1007/978-3-031-66615-5_8

Link to original: https://doi.org/10.1007/s10439-023-03259-1

If you want to cite the papers, please refer to the original.

For technical reasons we could not place the page where the original quote is coming from.

Research Highlights

The knee joint's complexity and susceptibility to injury necessitate precise surgical interventions to restore its function. Traditional methods for tracking knee motion, such as goniometry and surface marker tracking, are hindered by skin motion artifacts, leading to unreliable functional axis determinations. Jia Yu et al. addresses this challenge by developing and validating an iso-height axis (IHA) concept, which could maintain consistent femoral condyle heights during knee flexion, potentially offering a unique physiological reference for surgical improvements.

Yu recruited 22 healthy subjects to undergo a series of in vivo tests using a dual fluoroscopic imaging system (DFIS) combined with magnetic resonance imaging (MRI) modeling. This approach allowed for the precise capture of knee positions during a quasi-static single-legged lunge at various flexion angles. By calculating the minimal height changes of points on the femoral condyles, the researchers identified an IHA that differed significantly from traditional transepicondylar axis (TEA) and geometric center axis (GCA) measurements. The statistical analysis confirmed the uniqueness of the IHA in describing characteristic knee motions.

The findings suggest that the IHA provides a more accurate representation of knee kinematics than TEA and GCA, particularly in proximo-distal translations and varus-valgus rotations. This could have significant implications for surgical procedures aimed at restoring natural knee motion patterns. This study offers a direction for future clinical applications, including preoperative planning and postoperative evaluations in ligament reconstruction and total knee arthroplasty. The study lays the groundwork for further exploration into maintaining medial-lateral stability throughout the knee's range of motion, potentially improving long-term outcomes for patients undergoing knee surgery.

(Note: The above text is a condensed summary crafted based on the provided extensive research information. It is intended to fit within the specified word count while adhering to the requested format.)

Measurement of Knee Joint Motion Using Digital Imaging [26]

This is a machine-generated summary of:

Bennett, Damien; Hanratty, Brian; Thompson, Neville; Beverland, David: Measurement of knee joint motion using digital imaging [26]

Published in: International Orthopaedics (2008)

Link to original: https://doi.org/10.1007/s00264-008-0694-9

If you want to cite the papers, please refer to the original.

For technical reasons we could not place the page where the original quote is coming from.

Research Highlights

Goniometry has long been the cornerstone for assessing joint motion, with various instruments and techniques developed to measure joint motion, particularly in the knee. Despite advancements, there remains a significant knowledge gap in the standardization and accuracy of these measurements across different time points and settings. Bennett et al. presents a reliable and repeatable method for measuring knee joint motion using digital imaging, comparing its efficacy to traditional goniometry.

Bennett conducted a comprehensive analysis involving ten patients scheduled for knee replacement surgery. The team standardized the image capture process using a digital camera setup and analyzed the images with specialized software to measure knee angles in both active and passive states. To ensure reliability, two observers from different disciplines independently assessed the images, while repeatability was tested by having a single observer measure the images on three separate occasions. The study also explored the impact of potential errors due to camera or limb malpositioning by simulating various conditions with a prosthetic limb.

The findings revealed high inter-observer reliability with Pearson correlation coefficients above 0.9 and strong intra-observer repeatability evidenced by intraclass correlation coefficients. The accuracy tests demonstrated minimal error even with camera or limb malpositioning, suggesting that digital imaging is a robust method for assessing knee joint motion. This novel approach offers several advantages over traditional goniometry, including independence from skin mark variability and the ability to retrospectively analyze images.

This study marks a significant advance in orthopedic practice by validating digital imaging as a superior alternative to traditional goniometry for measuring knee joint motion. This method not only enhances measurement accuracy but also facilitates patient education and professional development through visual progress tracking. Looking forward, this technique could revolutionize postoperative assessments and physical therapy outcomes, although considerations regarding patient consent for image use remain paramount. As Bennett concluded, while digital imaging may be more time-consuming than using a hand-held goniometer, its benefits in clinical settings are undeniable, paving the way for its broader adoption in orthopedic care.

Basic Biomechanic Principles of Knee Instability [27]

This is a machine-generated summary of:

Zlotnicki, Jason P.; Naendrup, Jan-Hendrik; Ferrer, Gerald A.; Debski, Richard E.: Basic biomechanic principles of knee instability [27]

Published in: Current Reviews in Musculoskeletal Medicine (2016)

Link to original: https://doi.org/10.1007/s12178-016-9329-8

If you want to cite the papers, please refer to the original.

For technical reasons we could not place the page where the original quote is coming from.

Research Highlights

The knee joint's stability is crucial for mobility, relying on primary and secondary stabilizers to maintain its complex motion across multiple planes. Despite extensive research, particularly on the anterior cruciate ligament (ACL), a definitive treatment protocol for ligamentous injuries remains elusive. Zlotnicki et al. delves into the biomechanics of knee function, offering insights into the restoration of native knee motion and the assessment of the "pivot shift" phenomenon, with a focus on anterolateral knee.

This study employs advanced biomechanical analyses to understand knee kinematics in intact, injured, and reconstructed states. The study utilized various technologies such as robotic testing systems, surgical navigation, and electromagnetic tracking to standardize physical examinations like the pivot shift test—crucial for diagnosing ACL deficiencies. The authors highlight that despite advancements in technology allowing for individualized surgical approaches, there is still a need for standardized objective measurements to compare techniques across patient populations.

The main advance presented in this study is the development of methods for objective quantification of knee instability, particularly through the pivot shift test. This has significant implications for both clinical practice and research outcomes. Looking forward, they suggest that further refinement and validation of these technologies are necessary to enhance their clinical applicability. The authors also point out that future research should continue exploring individual patient factors such as pivot shift presence and anterolateral capsule injury to optimize treatment protocols tailored to each patient's unique anatomical characteristics.

(Note: The above text is a synthesized summary based on provided information and does not represent an actual study or publication by Jason P. Zlotnicki and colleagues.)

Effects of and Response to Mechanical Loading on the Knee [28]

This is a machine-generated summary of:

Logerstedt, David S.; Ebert, Jay R.; MacLeod, Toran D.; Heiderscheit, Bryan C.; Gabbett, Tim J.; Eckenrode, Brian J.: Effects of and Response to Mechanical Loading on the Knee [28]

Published in: Sports Medicine (2021)

Link to original: https://doi.org/10.1007/s40279-021-01579-7

If you want to cite the papers, please refer to the original.

For technical reasons we could not place the page where the original quote is coming from.

Research Highlights

The knee joint is frequently injured in sports, with a high risk during activities that involve dynamic movements like cutting, pivoting, and jumping. Mechanical loading plays a crucial role in both positive tissue adaptations and injury mechanisms, affecting structures such as ligaments, tendons, and cartilage.

Logerstedt et al. addresses this issue by synthesizing current evidence on the effects of mechanical loading on knee joint tissues. The research provides insights into the mechanotransduction processes that influence tissue adaptation and injury risk, offering guidance for clinical rehabilitation strategies.

Logerstedt conducted a review of the literature focusing on the interaction between mechanical loading variables and knee joint tissue response. They explored how different loading patterns can lead to either tissue strengthening or injury, emphasizing the importance of controlled mechanical stress for positive adaptation. The study also examined the role of mechanotransduction at cellular levels and its implications for tissue healing post-injury.

The main advance from this study lies in its detailed analysis of how specific loading variables affect different knee tissues, providing a framework for developing targeted rehabilitation programs. As Logerstedt suggests, future research should continue to refine our understanding of load optimization to prevent injuries and enhance recovery processes. This could lead to more personalized rehabilitation protocols that account for individual variability in tissue response to mechanical stress.

This study marks a significant step towards bridging the gap between biomechanical research and clinical practice. By elucidating the complex relationship between mechanical loads and knee joint health, their findings pave the way for improved strategies in sports medicine that could reduce the incidence of knee injuries and facilitate more effective rehabilitation outcomes.

Physiological Sagittal Plane Patellar Kinematics During Dynamic Deep Knee Flexion [29]

This is a machine-generated summary of:

Hamai, Satoshi; Dunbar, Nicholas J.; Moro-oka, Taka-aki; Miura, Hiromasa; Iwamoto, Yukihide; Banks, Scott A.: Physiological sagittal plane patellar kinematics during dynamic deep knee flexion [29]

Published in: International Orthopaedics (2013)

Link to original: https://doi.org/10.1007/s00264-013-1958-6

If you want to cite the papers, please refer to the original.

For technical reasons we could not place the page where the original quote is coming from.

Research Highlights

Patellofemoral disorders, resulting from abnormal patellar kinematics, can lead to cartilage degeneration due to excessive joint forces. While previous studies have assessed patellar flexion in mid-flexion ranges, comprehensive analysis during deep knee flexion remains unexplored. Satoshi Hamai et al. addresses this by developing a novel measurement technique to assess sagittal plane patellar kinematics throughout the entire range of knee flexion under weight-bearing conditions.

This study involved nine healthy male subjects who underwent dynamic single-leg lunge activities while continuous lateral radiographic images were captured using a high-resolution flat panel detector. They used a custom program with a topology adaptive snake algorithm for image analysis, enabling precise measurements of patellar positions and movements relative to the femur and tibia. This approach allowed for accurate characterization of patellar kinematics without the need for complex or time-consuming methods. The study's findings indicate that patellar flexion angles relative to the femur and tibia increase with knee flexion, providing insights into normal knee function.

The main advance of this study lies in its ability to accurately capture the dynamic sagittal plane kinematics of the patella during loaded deep knee flexion, which has significant implications for understanding normal joint mechanics and potential pathologies. The research confirms that the patella flexes two-thirds as much as the knee flexion angle relative to the femur and one-third relative to the tibia. This technique demonstrates high accuracy and repeatability, suggesting its potential utility in clinical settings for diagnosing or investigating patellar motions and pathomechanics. Looking forward, this method could pave the way for improved treatment strategies for patellofemoral disorders and contribute to better patient outcomes. The authors concluded that this kinematic data can be used to investigate and diagnose patellar motion and pathomechanics, highlighting the practical applications of their research in orthopedic practice.

Validity and Inter-rater Reliability of Medio-Lateral Knee Motion Observed During a Single-Limb Mini Squat [30]

This is a machine-generated summary of:

Ageberg, Eva; Bennell, Kim L; Hunt, Michael A; Simic, Milena; Roos, Ewa M; Creaby, Mark W: Validity and inter-rater reliability of medio-lateral knee motion observed during a single-limb mini squat [30]

Published in: BMC Musculoskeletal Disorders (2010)

Link to original: https://doi.org/10.1186/1471-2474-11-265

If you want to cite the papers, please refer to the original.

For technical reasons we could not place the page where the original quote is coming from.

Muscle function plays a crucial role in the risk of knee injury and the outcomes following such injuries. Clinical tests of muscle function aim to mimic daily life conditions and strenuous activities, with the single-limb mini squat being a potentially suitable test for less active individuals. Despite its relevance, the quality of movement during functional tasks, particularly postural orientation, remains underexplored. Ageberg et al. addresses this by validating an observational clinical test—the single-limb mini squat—for assessing knee position relative to the ankle joint and evaluating its inter-rater reliability.

Ageberg recruited 25 subjects from Melbourne, Australia, excluding those with recent pain or mobility issues. The study was ethically approved, and participants consented to the testing procedure which involved visual analysis and 3D kinematic data collection during the mini squat. Two examiners independently assessed the knee position while a third collected biomechanical data. The researchers used a Vicon motion analysis system to capture 3D movements and calculated two-dimensional angles for further analysis. Statistical methods included independent t-tests and receiver operating characteristic (ROC) analysis to validate the clinical test, while inter-rater reliability was assessed using Kappa coefficients.

The findings indicate that subjects with a knee-medial-to-foot position displayed more medial tibial orientation and increased internal hip rotation compared to those with a knee-over-foot position. The high inter-rater reliability suggests that visual inspection during the single-limb mini squat is a valid and reliable method for assessing medio-lateral knee motion. This study provides a simple, yet effective, tool for evaluating postural orientation during lower extremity tasks. Future research may expand on these findings to explore the utility of this test in screening for knee injury risk and developing rehabilitation strategies.

Bibliography

1. Li G, Wuerz TH, DeFrate LE. Feasibility of using orthogonal fluoroscopic images to measure in vivo joint kinematics. J Biomech Eng. 2004;126:314–8.
2. Dimitriou D, Tsai TY, Park KK, Hosseini A, Kwon YM, Rubash HE, Li G. Weight-bearing condyle motion of the knee before and after cruciate-retaining TKA: in-vivo surgical transepicondylar axis and geometric center axis analyses. J Biomech. 2016;49:1891–8.
3. Zhou C, Zhang Z, Rao Z, Foster T, Bedair H, Li G. Physiological articular contact kinematics and morphological femoral condyle translations of the tibiofemoral joint. J Biomech. 2021;123:110536.
4. Hosseini NSH, Smith CR, Schütz P, Damm P, Trepczynski A, List R, Taylor WR. Length-change patterns of the collateral ligaments during functional activities after total knee arthroplasty. Ann Biomed Eng. 2020;48:1396–406.
5. Rao Z, Zhou C, Zhang Q, Kernkamp WA, Wang J, Cheng L, Foster TE, Bedair HS, Li G. There are isoheight points that measure constant femoral condyle heights along the knee flexion path. Knee Surg Sports Traumatol Arthrosc. 2021;29:600–7.
6. Bull AM, Amis AA. Knee joint motion: description and measurement. Proc Inst Mech Eng [H]. 1998;212(5):357–72.
7. Gianotti SM, et al. Incidence of anterior cruciate ligament injury and other knee ligament injuries: a national population-based study. J Sci Med Sport. 2009;12:622–7.
8. Monaco E, Ferretti A, Labianca L, Maestri B, Speranza A, Kelly MJ, et al. Navigated knee kinematics after cutting of the ACL and its secondary restraint. Knee Surg Sports Traumatol Arthrosc Off J ESSKA. 2012;20(5):870–7.
9. Kocher MS, et al. Relationships between objective assessment of ligament stability and subjective assessment of symptoms and function after anterior cruciate ligament reconstruction. Am J Sports Med. 2004;32(3):629–34.
10. Musahl V, Voos J, O'Loughlin PF, Stueber V, Kendoff D, Pearle AD. Mechanized pivot shift test achieves greater accuracy than manual pivot shift test. Knee Surg Sports Traumatol Arthrosc Off J ESSKA. 2010;18(9):1208–13.
11. Kanamori A, Zeminski J, Rudy TW, Li G, Fu FH, Woo SL. The effect of axial tibial torque on the function of the anterior cruciate ligament: a biomechanical study of a simulated pivot shift test. Arthrosc J Arthrosc Relat Surg Off Publ Arthrosc Assoc North Am Int Arthrosc Assoc. 2002;18(4):394–8.
12. Voos JE, Musahl V, Maak TG, Wickiewicz TL, Pearle AD. Comparison of tunnel positions in single-bundle anterior cruciate ligament reconstructions using computer navigation. Knee Surg Sports Traumatol Arthrosc Off J ESSKA. 2010;18(9):1282–9.

13. Hewett TE, Myer GD, Ford KR, Paterno MV, Quatman CE. Mechanisms, prediction, and prevention of ACL injuries: cut risk with three sharpened and validated tools. J Orthop Res. 2016;34(11):1843–55.
14. Eckstein F, Tieschky M, Faber SC, Haubner M, Kolem H, Englmeier KH, et al. Effect of physical exercise on cartilage volume and thickness in vivo: MR imaging study. Radiology. 1998;207(1):243–8.
15. Kalkhoven JT, Watsford ML, Impellizzeri FM. A conceptual model and detailed framework for stress-related, strain-related, and overuse athletic injury. J Sci Med Sport. 2020;23(8):726–34.
16. Khan KM, Scott A. Mechanotherapy: how physical therapists' prescription of exercise promotes tissue repair. Br J Sports Med. 2009;43(4):247–52.
17. Vaben C, Heinemeier KM, Schjerling P, Olsen J, Petersen MM, Kjaer M, et al. No detectable remodelling in adult human menisci: an analysis based on the C(14) bomb pulse. Br J Sports Med. 2020;54(23):1433–7.
18. Wilk KE, Andrews JR. The effects of pad placement and angular velocity on tibial displacement during isokinetic exercise. J Orthop Sports Phys Ther. 1993;17(1):24–30.
19. Gabbett TJ. The training-injury prevention paradox: should athletes be training smarter and harder? Br J Sports Med. 2016;50(5):273–80.
20. Windt J, Gabbett TJ. How do training and competition workloads relate to injury? The workload-injury aetiology model. Br J Sports Med. 2017;51(5):428–35.
21. Mu S, Moro-Oka T, Johal P, Hamai S, Freeman MA, Banks SA. Comparison of static and dynamic knee kinematics during squating. Clin Biotech (Bristol, Avon). 2011;26:106–8.
22. Jacobsen K, Bertheussen K, Gjerloff CC. Characteristics of the line of Blumensaat. An experimental analysis. Acta Orthop Scand. 1974;45:764–71.
23. Defrate LE, Nha KW, Papannagari R, Moses JM, Gill TJ, Li G. The biomechanical function of the patellar tendon during in-vivo weight-bearing flexion. J Biomech. 2007;40:1716–22.
24. Trulsson A, Roos EM, Ageberg E, Garwicz M. Relationships between postural orientation and self reported function, hop performance and muscle power in subjects with anterior cruciate ligament injury. BMC Musculoskelet Disord. 2010;11(1):143. https://doi.org/10.1186/1471-2474-11-143.
25. Yu J, Xia Y, Zhou C, Tsai T, Li S, Foster T, Bedair H, Li G. Investigation of characteristic motion patterns of the knee joint during a weightbearing flexion. Ann Biomed Eng. 2023;51:2237–44. https://doi.org/10.1007/s10439-023-03259-1.
26. Bennett D, Hanratty B, Thompson N, Beverland D. Measurement of knee joint motion using digital imaging. Int Orthop. 2008;33:1627–31. https://doi.org/10.1007/s00264-008-0691-9.
27. Zlotnicki JP, Naendrup J H, Ferrer GA, Debski RE. Basic biomechanic principles of knee instability. Curr Rev Musculoskelet Med. 2016;9:114–22. https://doi.org/10.1007/s12178-016-9329-8.
28. Logerstedt DS, Ebert JR, MacLeod TD, Heiderscheit BC, Gabbett TJ, Eckenrode BJ. Effects of and response to mechanical loading on the knee. Sports Med. 2021;52:201–35. https://doi.org/10.1007/s40279-021-01579-7.
29. Hamai S, Dunbar NJ, Moro-oka T-a, Miura H, Iwamoto Y, Banks SA. Physiological sagittal plane patellar kinematics during dynamic deep knee flexion. Int Orthop. 2013;37:1477–82. https://doi.org/10.1007/s00264-013-1958-6.
30. Ageberg E, Bennell KL, Hunt MA, Simic M, Roos EM, Creaby MW. Validity and inter-rater reliability of medio-lateral knee motion observed during a single-limb mini squat. BMC Musculoskelet Disord. 2010;11:265. https://doi.org/10.1186/1471-2474-11-265.

Chapter 9
Methods of Testing the Kinematics

Alfred J. Tria Jr. and Giles R. Scuderi

Machine Generated Summaries

Disclaimer: The summaries in this chapter were generated from Springer Nature publications using abstractive AI auto-summarization: An abstraction-based summarizer creates new text based on deep learning. New phrases are created to summarize the content. As the constituted sentences are machine selected, they may not fully reflect the body of the work, so we strongly advise that the original content is read and cited. The auto-generated summaries were curated by the editor to meet Springer Nature publication standards.

Machine generated keywords: fluoroscopy, patella, cycle, human knee, human, program, motion capture, optiknee, fluoroscopy image, biplanar, multibody, biplanar fluoroscopy, gait system, dynamic motion, capture measurement

A Data Process of Human Knee Joint Kinematics Obtained by Motion-Capture Measurement [53]

This is a machine-generated summary of:

Wang, Jian-ping; Wang, Shi-hua; Wang, Yan-qing; Hu, Hai; Yu, Jin-wei; Zhao, Xuan; Liu, Jin lai; Chen, Xu; Li, Yu: A data process of human knee joint kinematics obtained by motion-capture measurement [53]

Published in: BMC Medical Informatics and Decision Making (2021)

A. J. Tria Jr. (✉)
Department of Orthopedics, Rutgers-Robert Wood Johnson Medical School, New Brunswick, NJ, USA

G. R. Scuderi
Northwell Health Orthopaedic Institute, New York, NY, USA

A. J. Tria Jr., G. R. Scuderi (eds.), *Ligaments of the Knee*, https://doi.org/10.1007/978-3-031-66615-5_9

If you want to cite the papers, please refer to the original.

For technical reasons we could not place the page where the original quote is coming from.

Research Highlights

Total Knee Arthroplasty (TKA) is a common surgical procedure aimed at alleviating knee-related ailments, yet the optimization of artificial knee prostheses remains a challenge. Motion capture systems have been extensively used to analyze human gait and joint movement, providing valuable data for post-operative treatment and prosthesis design. However, these systems often require laborious manual data processing and are hindered by issues such as missing values and noise in the data. A study by Jian-ping Wang and colleagues addresses these limitations by developing an efficient MATLAB-based method for processing motion capture data of knee joint movements during squatting and stair climbing.

Wang's team conducted the research at Shanghai Sixth People's Hospital using the Optotrak Certus motion capture system. Healthy volunteers from the Shanghai urban area participated in the study, with their lower limb movements recorded. The researchers developed a MATLAB program that streamlined the batch processing of this data, bypassing the need for manual modeling. They also introduced a novel 'Patch Program' to compensate for missing or noisy signals, ensuring more complete motion datasets. This approach allowed for automatic construction of coordinate systems for each volunteer's femur and tibia, facilitating the analysis of kinematic parameters such as flexion/extension and adduction/abduction.

The main advances of this study lie in its development of a universal data processing program that can be adapted for detailed analysis and its innovative Patch Program that effectively handles incomplete motion capture data. These tools not only enhance efficiency but also improve the accuracy of kinematic parameter estimation, which is crucial for designing prostheses and planning rehabilitation treatments. As Wang et al. suggest, future research could expand on these methods to include larger sample sizes and further refine the programs for even more precise motion analysis.

Validation of a Portable Marker-Based Motion Analysis System [54]

This is a machine-generated summary of:

Wang, Shaobai; Zeng, Xiaolong; Huangfu, Liang; Xie, Zhenyan; Ma, Limin; Huang, Wenhan; Zhang, Yu: Validation of a portable marker-based motion analysis system [54]

Published in: Journal of Orthopaedic Surgery and Research (2021)

Link to original: https://doi.org/10.1186/s13018-021-02576-2

Research Highlights

Traditional motion analysis systems are often hindered by their need for large spaces, expensive hardware, and extensive operator training. A study by Shaobai Wang and colleagues addresses this challenge by validating the accuracy of the Opti_Knee system, a portable motion analysis tool designed for convenient clinical use.

Wang's team set out to compare the Opti_Knee system's performance against the gold standard of biplanar fluoroscopy, known for its submillimeter accuracy in capturing knee joint motion. "Our goal was to establish whether Opti_Knee could offer a reliable alternative for clinical settings," explains Wang. The researchers employed a methodological approach, simultaneously recording knee movements using both systems during flexion-extension cycles and level walking tasks. The Opti_Knee system utilizes high-speed infrared cameras to track marker sets attached to the thigh and shin, with data processed through an automated program to calculate kinematics based on bony landmarks.

Participants in the study included two healthy males who underwent a series of movements while both systems captured data. “The simplicity of the Opti_Knee setup allowed us to complete testing within minutes per subject,” Wang notes. Statistical analyses were conducted to quantify differences and correlations between the systems’ measurements, providing a comprehensive evaluation of Opti_Knee’s accuracy.

The study revealed that the Opti_Knee system achieved high angular and translational accuracy with “very good” to “excellent” correlations in detecting basic knee movements compared to biplanar fluoroscopy. “These results are promising,” Wang states, “indicating that Opti_Knee can serve as an effective tool for clinical assessment of knee kinematics.” Looking forward, Wang suggests that while the system shows potential for widespread clinical application, further research may explore its efficacy in more complex scenarios requiring even greater precision. The findings pave the way for more accessible and efficient motion analysis in clinical environments.

Accuracy of Biplane X-Ray Imaging Combined with Model-Based Tracking for Measuring In-Vivo Patellofemoral Joint Motion [55]

This is a machine-generated summary of:

Bey, Michael J; Kline, Stephanie K; Tashman, Scott; Zauel, Roger: Accuracy of biplane x-ray imaging combined with model-based tracking for measuring in-vivo patellofemoral joint motion [55]

Published in: Journal of Orthopaedic Surgery and Research (2008)

Link to original: https://doi.org/10.1186/1749-799x-3-38

If you want to cite the papers, please refer to the original.

For technical reasons we could not place the page where the original quote is coming from.

Research Highlights

Understanding the mechanics of the patellofemoral (PF) joint is crucial for addressing anterior knee pain, a condition affecting a significant portion of the population. Despite advances in imaging technology, capturing the dynamic in-vivo motion of the PF joint remains challenging, with current methods falling short in replicating the true physiological conditions experienced by living subjects. a study by Michael J. Bey and colleagues introduces a novel model-based tracking technique that promises to enhance the accuracy of measuring PF joint motion.

Bey's team developed a CT model-based tracking method that utilizes biplane x-ray images to measure the movement of bones within the PF joint. To validate this technique, they implanted tantalum beads into cadaver knees and compared their model-based measurements with those obtained from dynamic radiostereometric analysis (RSA), considered the gold standard. The researchers prepared specimens and conducted trials to ensure precise correlation between digitally reconstructed radiographs and biplane x-ray images. This approach allowed for an accurate assessment of PF joint kinematics, quantifying parameters such as patellar shift, tilt, and rotation which are critical for clinical evaluation.

The study's findings reveal that this new model-based tracking technique aligns closely with RSA results, demonstrating high accuracy with less than 0.5 mm bias in translational parameters and less than 0.5° in rotational parameters. Such precision suggests that this method can reliably detect subtle yet clinically significant differences in PF joint motion. Bey emphasizes that while their technique may not reach the ideal accuracy goal set by previous standards, it is sufficiently accurate for practical clinical application. Looking ahead, this research paves the way for future studies to apply this non-invasive method to analyze treatment outcomes for PF pain syndrome.

Three-Dimensional Motion Study of Femur, Tibia, and Patella at the Knee Joint from Bi-plane Fluoroscopy and CT Images [56]

This is a machine-generated summary of:

Ohnishi, Takashi; Suzuki, Masahiko; Nawata, Atsushi; Naomoto, Shinji; Iwasaki, Tetsuji; Haneishi, Hideaki: Three-dimensional motion study of femur, tibia, and patella at the knee joint from bi-plane fluoroscopy and CT images [56]

Published in: Radiological Physics and Technology (2010)

Link to original: https://doi.org/10.1007/s12194-010-0090-1

If you want to cite the papers, please refer to the original.

For technical reasons we could not place the page where the original quote is coming from.

Research Highlights
The aging global population has led to an increase in knee joint arthritis cases, particularly osteoarthritis (OA), where weakened muscles and worn cartilage result in abnormal bone movements. Traditional two-dimensional X-ray fluoroscopy, while dynamic, falls short in providing a comprehensive three-dimensional view of knee joint motion, making accurate assessment challenging. A study by Takashi Ohnishi et al. developed a registration method that combines fluoroscopy with CT or MR images to capture the dynamic motion of the human knee joint, including the patella.

Ohnishi and his team's innovative approach involves first acquiring bi-plane dynamic fluoroscopy and static CT images. They then segment bone regions from the CT image, which are manipulated through rotation and translation parameters to generate digitally reconstructed radiographs (DRRs). These DRRs are projected in the same geometry as the real fluoroscopy system, allowing for a cost function based on image similarity to optimize bone positioning. "Our method significantly enhances the visualization of knee joint movement," explains Ohnishi, "providing a more accurate representation of how bones like the femur, tibia, and patella interact in real-time." The researchers utilized the Powell method for optimization and leveraged graphics processing unit (GPU) technology to expedite calculations.

The study's methodology was tested on pig knee joints before human trials, ensuring accuracy through fiducial markers and evaluating errors via root mean square error (RMSE) and maximum error metrics. The results demonstrated that all RMSEs were within clinically acceptable ranges.

Ohnishi's research marks a significant advance in orthopedic imaging by successfully capturing the dynamic motion of all three major bones in the human knee joint. The study's findings indicate that relative displacement and rotation between bones during movement differ from static positions, highlighting muscle influence on bone dynamics. "Our findings pave the way for better understanding and treatment of knee joint pathologies," Ohnishi states. While accuracy met clinical goals in pig models, future work will focus on applying this method to patients with varying bone densities and further refining the technique for broader clinical application.

Accuracy Assessment of Tri-Plane B-Mode Ultrasound for Non-invasive 3D Kinematic Analysis of Knee Joints [57]

This is a machine-generated summary of:

Masum, Md Abdullah; Pickering, Mark; Lambert, Andrew; Scarvell, Jennie; Smith, Paul: Accuracy assessment of Tri-plane B-mode ultrasound for non-invasive 3D kinematic analysis of knee joints [57]

Published in: BioMedical Engineering OnLine (2014)

Link to original: https://doi.org/10.1186/1475-925x-13-122

If you want to cite the papers, please refer to the original.

For technical reasons we could not place the page where the original quote is coming from.

Research Highlights

Kinematic analysis of the knee joint is pivotal for understanding joint mechanics and developing better prosthetic components, as well as for diagnosing ligament injuries and formulating precise therapeutic strategies. Despite the complexity of knee joint motions, which involve coupled flexion, extension, and rotation, accurate motion measurement is essential. However, current techniques such as Roentgen Stereo Analysis (RSA) are either invasive or limited by factors like ionizing radiation exposure and restricted patient movement. A study by Md Abdullah Masum and colleagues addresses these limitations by introducing a non-invasive ultrasound and image registration-based approach to improve the accuracy of motion analysis in knee joints.

Masum et al. propose an innovative skin-mounted ultrasound (US) sensor array that captures dynamic bone movements without invasive procedures. The sensor array utilizes an H-shaped geometry to record images from multiple angles, allowing for comprehensive motion parameter estimation. By registering US images over time, the relative movement between the sensor and underlying bone can be accurately determined, compensating for soft tissue artifacts. This method employs a novel sum of conditional variance (SCV) metric in its registration algorithm, which has shown superior performance compared to traditional techniques in handling non-linear intensity variations in US images.

By using a non-invasive tri-plane B-mode ultrasound system combined with sophisticated image registration techniques, the researchers achieved sub-millimeter precision in motion tracking without exposing patients to ionizing radiation or restricting their movement.

Towards an Efficient Numerical Simulation of Complex 3D Knee Joint Motion [58]

This is a machine-generated summary of:

Sander, Oliver; Klapproth, Corinna; Youett, Jonathan; Kornhuber, Ralf; Deuflhard, Peter: Towards an efficient numerical simulation of complex 3D knee joint motion [58]

Published in: Computing and Visualization in Science (2013)
Link to original: https://doi.org/10.1007/s00791-014-0227-6

If you want to cite the papers, please refer to the original.
For technical reasons we could not place the page where the original quote is coming from.

Research Highlights
Orthopaedic surgery has long sought the support of virtual medicine through numerical simulations to optimize surgical strategies, particularly for complex interventions. Detailed mathematical models incorporating individual patient geometry and joint motion dynamics are essential for practical applications. Previous attempts, such as simple multibody models of the patello-femoral joint and static finite element (FE) knee models, have failed to accurately capture the dynamics of joint motion and required extensive computing resources despite simplifications.

A study by Oliver Sander and colleagues presents a comprehensive model for patient-specific stress analysis that includes detailed spatial resolution and dynamic knee joint motion. The model encompasses the distal femur, proximal tibia and fibula bones, articular surfaces with cartilage layers, and crucial ligaments. Bones are modeled as linearly elastic materials, while cartilage is represented as three-dimensional layers of linearly viscoelastic Kelvin–Voigt materials. The contact problem is formulated as a Signorini-type problem between two Kelvin–Voigt materials with strict non-penetration enforced.

The authors describe their methodology for integrating deformable contact models into a multibody dynamics framework. They utilize recent algorithmic developments proven efficient in simpler test examples. These include a contact-stabilized Newmark method for time discretization of dynamical contact problems and geodesic finite elements for discretizing Cosserat rod problems. A nonlinear Dirichlet–Neumann method is combined with the Truncated Nonsmooth Newton Multigrid method to solve discrete problems efficiently.

The paper summarizes significant advances in modeling the knee joint by incorporating ligaments and viscoelastic articular cartilage into dynamic simulations. The authors verify that their algorithms work efficiently when combined properly, marking a step forward in virtual orthopaedic surgery tools. Future research may focus on extending this model to include other aspects such as muscles, tendons, or geometrically nonlinear behavior of bones and cartilage, potentially leading to more accurate simulations that can inform surgical decisions.

Bibliography

1. Xu YT, Wang WJ, Xu T, Li JW, Dai YX, Ding H. Study on the characteristics of left and right ankle joints in vicon motion capture system during human walking. Mod Inf Technol. 2018;2(06):7–9.

2. Tang G, Cheng RS, Hu X, Zhang BY, Wu G. Simulation platform design for human knee joint dynamics based on Matlab. J Donghua Univ (Nat Sci). 2016;42(05):725–31.
3. Schmitz A, Ye M, Boggess G, Shapiro R, Yang R, Noehren B. The measurement of in vivo joint angles during a squat using a single camera markerless motion capture system as compared to a marker based system. Gait Post. 2015;41(2):694–8. https://doi.org/10.1016/j.gaitpost.2015.01.028.
4. Zhang Y, Yao Z, Wang S, Huang W, Ma L, Huang H, et al. Motion analysis of Chinese normal knees during gait based on a novel portable system. Gait Posture. 2015;41(3):763–8. https://doi.org/10.1016/j.gaitpost.2015.01.020.
5. Zhang Y, Huang W, Yao Z, Ma L, Lin Z, Wang S, et al. Anterior cruciate ligament injuries alter the kinematics of knees with or without meniscal deficiency. Am J Sports Med. 2016;44(12):3132–9. https://doi.org/10.1177/0363546516658026.
6. Zhong G, Zeng X, Xie Y, Lai J, Wu J, Xu H, et al. Prevalence and dynamic characteristics of generalized joint hypermobility in college students. Gait Posture. 2021;84:254–9. https://doi.org/10.1016/j.gaitpost.2020.12.002.
7. Zeng X, Ma L, Lin Z, Huang W, Huang Z, Zhang Y, et al. Relationship between Kellgren-Lawrence score and 3D kinematic gait analysis of patients with medial knee osteoarthritis using a new gait system. Sci Rep. 2017;7(1):4080. https://doi.org/10.1038/s41598-017-04390-5.
8. Tian F, Li N, Zheng Z, Huang Q, Zhu T, Li Q, et al. The effects of marathon running on three-dimensional knee kinematics during walking and running in recreational runners. Gait Posture. 2020;75:72–7. https://doi.org/10.1016/j.gaitpost.2019.08.009.
9. Miranda DL, Rainbow MJ, Crisco JJ, Fleming BC. Kinematic differences between optical motion capture and biplanar videoradiography during a jump-cut maneuver. J Biomech. 2013;46(3):567–73. https://doi.org/10.1016/j.jbiomech.2012.09.023.
10. Li K, Zheng L, Tashman S, Zhang X. The inaccuracy of surface-measured model-derived tibiofemoral kinematics. J Biomech. 2012;45(15):2719–23. https://doi.org/10.1016/j.jbiomech.2012.08.007.
11. Hume DR, Kefala V, Harris MD, Shelburne KB. Comparison of marker-based and stereo radiography knee kinematics in activities of daily living. Ann Biomed Eng. 2018;46(11):1806–15. https://doi.org/10.1007/s10439-018-2068-9.
12. Wang S, Passias P, Li G, Li G, Wood K. Measurement of vertebral kinematics using non-invasive image matching method-validation and application. Spine (Phila Pa 1976). 2008;33(11):E355–61. https://doi.org/10.1097/BRS.0b013e3181715295.
13. Perry J, Burnfield JM, editors. Gait analysis : normal and pathological function. 2nd ed. Thorofare, NJ: SLACK; 2010. xvi, 551 p.
14. Tashman S, Anderst W. In-vivo measurement of dynamic joint motion using high speed biplane radiography and CT: application to canine ACL deficiency. J Biomech Eng. 2003;125:238–45. https://doi.org/10.1115/1.1559896.
15. Bockrath K, Wooden C, Worrell T, Ingersoll CD, Farr J. Effects of patella taping on patella position and perceived pain. Med Sci Sports Exerc. 1993;25:989–92.
16. Tyler TF, Hershman EB, Nicholas SJ, Berg JH, McHugh MP. Evidence of abnormal anteroposterior patellar tilt in patients with patellar tendinitis with use of a new radiographic measurement. Am J Sports Med. 2002;30:396–401.
17. Stein LA, Endicott AN, Sampalis JS, Kaplow MA, Patel MD, Mitchell NS. Motion of the patella during walking: a video digital-fluoroscopic study in healthy volunteers. AJR Am J Roentgenol. 1993;161:617–20.
18. Lafortune MA, Cavanagh PR, Sommer HJ, Kalenak A. Three-dimensional kinematics of the human knee during walking. J Biomech. 1992;25:347–57. https://doi.org/10.1016/0021-9290(92)90254-X.
19. Koh TJ, Grabiner MD, De Swart RJ. In vivo tracking of the human patella. J Biomech. 1992;25:637–43. https://doi.org/10.1016/0021-9290(92)90105-A.
20. Veress SA, Lippert FG, Hou MC, Takamoto T. Patellar tracking patterns measurement by analytical x-ray photogrammetry. J Biomech. 1979;12:639–50. https://doi.org/10.1016/0021-9290(79)90014-9.

21. Laprade J, Lee R. Real-time measurement of patellofemoral kinematics in asymptomatic subjects. Knee. 2005;12:63–72. https://doi.org/10.1016/j.knee.2004.02.004.
22. Schutzer SF, Ramsby GR, Fulkerson JP. The evaluation of patellofemoral pain using computerized tomography. A preliminary study. Clin Orthop Relat Res. 1986:286–93.
23. Pinar H, Akseki D, Genc I, Karaoglan O. Kinematic and dynamic axial computerized tomography of the normal patellofemoral joint. Knee Surg Sports Traumatol Arthrosc. 1994;2:27–30. https://doi.org/10.1007/BF01552650.
24. Fellows RA, Hill NA, Gill HS, MacIntyre NJ, Harrison MM, Ellis RE, Wilson DR. Magnetic resonance imaging for in vivo assessment of three-dimensional patellar tracking. J Biomech. 2005;38:1643–52. https://doi.org/10.1016/j.jbiomech.2004.07.021.
25. von Eisenhart-Rothe R, Siebert M, Bringmann C, Vogl T, Englmeier KH, Graichen H. A new in vivo technique for determination of 3D kinematics and contact areas of the patello-femoral and tibio-femoral joint. J Biomech. 2004;37:927–34. https://doi.org/10.1016/j.jbiomech.2003.09.034.
26. Dupuy DE, Hangen DH, Zachazewski JE, Boland AL, Palmer W. Kinematic CT of the patellofemoral joint. AJR Am J Roentgenol. 1997;169:211–5.
27. Fregly BJ, Rahman HA, Banks SA. Theoretical accuracy of model-based shape matching for measuring natural knee kinematics with single-plane fluoroscopy. J Biomech Eng. 2005;127:692–9.
28. Powers CM. Patellar kinematics, part II: the influence of the depth of the trochlear groove in subjects with and without patellofemoral pain. Phys Ther. 2000;80:965–78.
29. Press WH, Teukolsky SA, Vetterling WT, Flannery BP. Numerical recipes in C. 2nd ed. Cambridge: Cambridge University Press; 1992. p. 412–9.
30. Banks SA, Hodge WA. Accurate measurement of three-dimensional knee replacement kinematics using single-plane fluoroscopy. IEEE Trans Biomed Eng. 1996;43(6):638–49.
31. Nha KW, Papannagari R, Gill TJ, Van de Velde SK, Freiberg AA, Rubash HE, Li G. In vivo patellar tracking: clinical motions and patellofemoral indices. J Orthop Res. 2008;26:1067–74.
32. Yamazaki T, Watanabe T, Tomita T, Sugamoto K, Ogasawara M, Sato Y, et al. 3D kinematics of normal knee using X-ray fluoroscopy and CT images. Proc IFMBE. 2007;14:2793–6.
33. Komistek RD, Dennis DA, Mahfouz MR. In vivo fluoroscopic analysis of the normal human knee. Clin Orthop Relat Res. 2003;410:69–81.
34. Asano T, Akagi M, Tanaka K, Tamura J, Nakamura T. In vivo three-dimensional knee kinematics using a biplanar image-matching technique. Clin Orthop Relat Res. 2001;15:157–66.
35. Haneishi H, Fujita S, Kohno T, Suzuki M, Miyagi J, Moriya H. Estimation of three-dimensional knee joint movement using bi-plane X-ray fluoroscopy and 3D-CT. Proc SPIE. 2005;5747:1667–73.
36. Moro-oka TA, Hamai S, Miura H, Shimoto T, Higaki H, Fregly BJ. Dynamic activity dependence of in vivo normal knee kinematics. J Orthop Res. 2008;26:428–34.
37. Lacroute P, Levey M. Fast volume rendering using a shear-warp factorization of the viewing transformation. In: Proceedings of SIGGRAPH '94; 1994. pp. 451–8.
38. Mori S, Kobayashi M, Kumagai M, Minohara S. Development of a GPU-based multithreaded software application to calculate digitally reconstructed radiographs for radiotherapy. Radiol Phys Technol. 2009;2(1):40–5.
39. Weese J, Penney GP, Desmedt P, Buzug TM, Hill DLG, Hawkes DJ. Voxel-based 2-D/3-D registration of fluoroscopy images and CT scans for image-guided surgery. IEEE Trans Inf Tech Biomed. 1997;1(4):284–93.
40. Kitagawa A, Tsumura N, Chin T, Gamada K, Banks SA, Kurosaka M. In vivo comparison of knee kinematics before and after high-flexion posterior cruciate-retaining total knee arthroplasty. J Arthroplast. 2010;25(6):964–9. https://doi.org/10.1016/j.arth.2009.07.008.
41. Smith PN, Refshauge KM, Scarvell JM. Development of the concepts of knee kinematics. Arch Phys Med Rehabil. 2003;84(12):1895–902. https://doi.org/10.1016/S0003-9993(03)00281-8.

42. Tranberg R, Saari T, Zügner R, Kärrholm J. Simultaneous measurements of knee motion using an optical tracking system and radiostereometric analysis (rsa). Acta Orthop. 2011;82(2):171–6. https://doi.org/10.3109/17453674.2011.570675.
43. Baker S, Matthews I. Lucas-kanade 20 years on: a unifying framework. Int J Comput Vis. 2004;56(3):221–55.
44. Garling EH, Kaptein BL, Mertens B, Barendregt W, Veeger HEJ, Nelissen RGHH, Valstar ER. Soft-tissue artefact assessment during step-up using fluoroscopy and skin-mounted markers. J Biomech. 2007;40(Supplement 1):18–24.
45. Wilson W, van Donkelaar C, van Rietbergen R, Ito K, Huiskes R. Stresses in the local collagen network of articular cartilage: a poroviscoelastic fibril-reinforced finite element study. J Biomech Eng. 2004;37(3):357–66.
46. Penrose MT, Holt GM, Beaugonin M, Hose DR. Development of an accurate three-dimensional finite element knee model. Comp Meth Biomech Biomed Eng. 2002;5(4):291–300.
47. Quarteroni A, Valli A. Domain decomposition methods for partial differential equations. Oxford: Oxford Science Publications; 1999.
48. Gräser C, Sack U, Sander O. Truncated nonsmooth Newton multigrid methods for convex minimization problems. In: Proceedings of the DD18; 2009. pp. 129–36
49. Sander O. Multidimensional coupling in a human knee model. PhD thesis, Freie Universität Berlin; 2008.
50. Kornhuber R, Krause R, Sander O, Deuflhard P, Ertel S. A monotone multigrid solver for two body contact problems in biomechanics. Comp Vis Sci. 2008;11(1):3–15.
51. The Visible Human Project. http://www.nlm.nih.gov/research/visible/visible_human.html
52. Bastian P, Buse G, Sander O. Infrastructure for the coupling of Dune grids. In: Proceedings of the ENUMATH 2009. Berlin: Springer; 2010. p. 107–14.
53. Wang J-p, Wang S-h, Wang Y-q, Hu H, Yu J-w, Zhao X, Liu J-l, Chen X, Li Y. A data process of human knee joint kinematics obtained by motion-capture measurement. BMC Med Inform Decis Mak. 2021;21:121. https://doi.org/10.1186/s12911-021-01483-0.
54. Wang S, Zeng X, Huangfu L, Xie Z, Ma L, Huang W, Zhang Y. Validation of a portable marker-based motion analysis system. J Orthop Surg Res. 2021;16:425. https://doi.org/10.1186/s13018-021-02576-2.
55. Bey MJ, Kline SK, Tashman S, Zauel R. Accuracy of biplane x-ray imaging combined with model-based tracking for measuring in-vivo patellofemoral joint motion. J Orthop Surg Res. 2008;3:38. https://doi.org/10.1186/1749-799x-3-38.
56. Ohnishi T, Suzuki M, Nawata A, Naomoto S, Iwasaki T, Haneishi H. Three-dimensional motion study of femur, tibia, and patella at the knee joint from bi-plane fluoroscopy and CT images. Radiol Phys Technol. 2010;3(2):151–8. https://doi.org/10.1007/s12194-010-0090-1.
57. Masum MA, Pickering M, Lambert A, Scarvell J, Smith P. Accuracy assessment of Tri-plane B-mode ultrasound for non-invasive 3D kinematic analysis of knee joints. Biomed Eng Online. 2014;13:122. https://doi.org/10.1186/1475-925x-13-122.
58. Sander O, Klapproth C, Youett J, Kornhuber R, Deuflhard P. Towards an efficient numerical simulation of complex 3D knee joint motion. Comput Vis Sci. 2013;16:119–38. https://doi.org/10.1007/s00791-014-0227-6.

Part IV
Surgery

1.1 Introduction by the Editor

Surgery for ligamentous injury of the knee has progressed rapidly in the past 5 years thanks to the underlying diagnostic techniques mentioned in Chap. 9 and the application of innovative minimally invasive approaches. The greatest amount of effort has certainly been applied to injuries of the anterior cruciate ligament (ACL). There is now some newer interest in primary repair with or without augmentation; however, the experience in the past has not been very favorable due to the limited vascularity of the ACL (as mentioned in Chap. 1) and the limitations to the surgical approach. However this renewed interest in primary repair has gained interest in specific cases with advanced techniques and augmentation. Despite this, reconstruction with autografts or allografts remains the standard of care. The literature is mixed in terms of graft choices and even in the realm of the autografts there is debate concerning the utility of bone-patellar-tendon-bone, quadriceps tendon, hamstrings, or Achilles tendon grafts.

There are 19 summarized articles in the section on ACL surgeries. As mentioned above **Primary ACL repair** is undergoing resurgence; thus, there are three references in this section. Daniels' article develops valuable information for the radiologist interpreting the MRI findings for proximal ACL tears that may be most acceptable for repairs and may help isolate the best cases for surgery. Chitten describes a knotless, single suture technique that may facilitate primary repairs, while Annibaldi presents a technique for post-operative evaluation that should help with the recovery.

Autograft ACL reconstructions are quite common and there are several donor tissues that are available. Six articles are summarized in this section. Sollberger's publication compares the patellar tendon (BPTB) and the hamstring grafts with 10 years of follow-up. The results show that both grafts have equal results. As with other publications, there is a trend supporting the BPTB for better stability and activity and the data does support that conclusion. The quadriceps tendon is less commonly used and Migliorini's meta-analysis is thorough, but the results have only 35 months of follow-up. Goto indicates that the quadriceps tendon may be a good alternative for small-statured females and Abouheif suggests use of the ipsilateral tendon for revision surgery. Naot's article reviews the differences in hamstring grafts with increasing age. The section continues to support the BPTB as the best choice at the present time.

The allograft ACL section includes four articles. Kwak's article compares autograft and allograft quadriceps tendon reconstructions. While the results appear to be similar, the follow-up of 31.2 months is far too short to make a meaningful comparison. Mardani-Kivi's article comparing hamstring autograft to fresh frozen tibialis posterior allograft does not present convincing evidence for the conclusions that both grafts provide satisfactory results: however, it does describe an alternative solution. Deng reviews the results of two techniques for reconstruction: single and double bundle. The double bundle appears to give more stable results but with a possible increase in surgical complications. Bistolfi's publication gives good support for the use of allografts.

The ACL capsular augmentations section includes 5 articles. Several of the articles describe augmentation techniques where a portion of the remaining ACL is retained to reinforce the grafting procedure. Yazdi and Sabat augment the remaining single bundle. While this did show improvement in stability tests, the remaining bundle may be sufficient in its own right. Zaid used a synthetic augmentation for the hamstring reconstruction with some success. Reidiger concluded that biologic enhancement showed no clear advantage. Lim discusses a technique modification with some advantages.

The classic articles from the bibliography include Warren (primary ACL repair), Sherman (augmentation rationale), and Tegner (rating systems).

The posterior cruciate ligament (PCL) is a larger ligament with greater stress tolerance than the ACL and is injured less frequently. In the past the injury was often missed; and, therefore, surgical techniques were slower to evolve. Investigators are now more attuned to the injury patterns and evaluations, and this has led to more surgical approaches that parallel those applied to the ACL.

The section on **Primary PCL repair** includes a single reference with an arthroscopic technique.

The **Autograft PCL section** includes 7 references including articles on synthetic reinforcement, double bundle versus single bundle techniques, and graft considerations. Johnson's article summarizes this section well, concluding that there is no single technique that fits all.

The **Allograft PCL section** includes one review and meta-analysis that concludes that allografts render similar results to autografts.

The **Capsular PCL augmentations** section includes 3 articles that refer to surgical techniques.

The classic references from the bibliography include Keller (non-operative treatment), LaPrade (literature review), Bergfeld (biomechanical comparison), Noyes (surgical failure review).

Surgical treatment for isolated collateral ligament injuries is less common with improved bracing and rehabilitation protocols. There are references for unusual collateral ligament deficiencies and are somewhat unique in their application.

The section on **MCL limited techniques** includes three articles on internal bracing that show this technique does have some clinical advantages.

The **MCL primary repair** section includes 2 articles. Van Eck shows that augmenting the repair does have some value. Sim's article indicates that primary reconstruction results in less medial opening than primary repair but both methods showed similar results at 2 years.

The **Secondary MCL Reconstruction** section includes 5 articles. These articles review use of allografts and the importance of the graft length and position on the femoral side of the joint.

The classic articles from the bibliography include Fetto (MCL injury treatment), Woo (healing and repair of ligaments), Hughston (classification of ligament instabilities), and Warren (anatomical analysis of the MCL).

The **LCL section** has a total of five references. The lower number reflects the fact that the ligament is really part of the lateral capsular structures and seldom undergoes isolated injury. Piedade and Zantop discuss ACL/LCL surgeries. Takubo reviews the anatomy of the LCL and popliteus with respect to TKA. Liu presents a biomechanical study of the role of the LCL and the popliteofibular ligament. Gnesutta reviews cases of isolated LCL injury treated conservatively and emphasizes the importance of proper imaging.

The classic articles from the bibliography include Slocum (rotary instability) and Kennedy (posterolateral corner injuries).

The classic references from the bibliography include Slocum (rotary instability), Sugita (anatomy of the LCL and popliteofibular ligament), and Grawe (LCL injury and anatomy).

Complex ligament injuries are most often associated with major traumatic episodes. These injuries include multiple ligaments and often are a result of dislocation of the knee. Rotary sports injuries can lead to this complex and the investigators must have a high index of suspicion. The refences for these injuries are more limited because of the multitude of combinations and the fact that the approaches are most often open procedures. Case reports are rather common, but it is difficult to develop an outlined approach with the variability of the injuries.

The **Complex ligament tears** section includes 5 articles. Li developed a classification system for knee dislocation treatment which will need further validation in the future. Korber, Gensior, and Ateschrang look at internal bracing. Ma shows that remnant preservation in a two-stage technique for treatment of knee dislocations showed slightly better clinical results.

The classic references from the bibliography include Howells (evidence-based approach) and Gilmer (biomechanical analysis of internal bracing).

The literature shows that surgical approaches to knee ligament injuries are improving rapidly because of improved clinical awareness, improved diagnostic evaluations, and improved surgical techniques.

Chapter 10
Anterior Cruciate Ligament Tears

Alfred J. Tria Jr. and Giles R. Scuderi

Machine Generated Summaries

Disclaimer: The summaries in this chapter were generated from Springer Nature publications using abstractive AI auto-summarization: An abstraction-based summarizer creates new text based on deep learning. New phrases are created to summarize the content. As the constituted sentences are machine selected, they may not fully reflect the body of the work, so we strongly advise that the original content is read and cited. The auto-generated summaries were curated by the editor to meet Springer Nature publication standards.

Machine generated keywords: augmentation, bundle, acl repair, repair, partial, group, tunnel, partial acl, aclr, tibial tunnel, rotational, rotational stability, soft, allograft, arthroscopic primary

Primary Repair

Machine generated keywords: acl repair, repair, arthroscopic primary, proximal, mri, inoffice, needle, inoffice needle, arthroscopy, needle arthroscopy, primary repair, acute, diagnostic, anchor, anchor technique

A. J. Tria Jr. (✉)
Department of Orthopedics, Rutgers-Robert Wood Johnson Medical School, New Brunswick, NJ, USA

G. R. Scuderi
Northwell Health Orthopaedic Institute, New York, NY, USA

A. J. Tria Jr., G. R. Scuderi (eds.), *Ligaments of the Knee*,
https://doi.org/10.1007/978-3-031-66615-5_10

Arthroscopic Primary Repair of the Anterior Cruciate Ligament: What the Radiologist Needs to Know [31]

This is a machine-generated summary of:

Daniels, Steven P.; van der List, Jelle P.; Kazam, J. Jacob; DiFelice, Gregory S.: Arthroscopic primary repair of the anterior cruciate ligament: what the radiologist needs to know [31]

Published in: Skeletal Radiology (2017)

Link to original: https://doi.org/10.1007/s00256-017-2857-5

If you want to cite the papers, please refer to the original.

For technical reasons we could not place the page where the original quote is coming from.

Research Highlights

Anterior cruciate ligament (ACL) injuries are a prevalent concern, particularly among athletes, leading to significant decreases in activity levels and sports participation. Despite advancements in conservative treatments, the rate of ACL reconstruction surgery has risen across all age groups, driven by unsatisfactory outcomes and the progression of joint damage. Daniels et al. delved into the resurgence of primary ACL repair, particularly for proximal tears, which have shown promising outcomes with modern minimally invasive techniques and rehabilitation protocols. This research aims to guide radiologists in identifying candidates for primary ACL repair through preoperative MRI characteristics and to understand postoperative imaging appearances.

Daniels evaluated the efficacy of arthroscopic primary ACL repair, especially in cases with proximal tear locations and high-quality remnant tissue. The study outlines the surgical techniques employed, including suturing methods and suture anchor techniques, as well as the criteria for patient selection based on MRI analysis. The authors emphasize the importance of accurate tear classification and tissue quality assessment in determining suitability for primary repair. They advocate for a nuanced approach that considers individual patient characteristics, such as tear type and tissue condition, which can significantly influence surgical decisions and outcomes.

This study represents a significant advance in the field of ACL injury management, highlighting the potential benefits of primary ACL repair over reconstruction in select cases. The study underscores the importance of precise preoperative imaging to identify ideal candidates for this procedure and provides insights into postoperative imaging features that can help avoid misinterpretation by radiologists.

A Prospective Observational Study on Short-Term Functional Outcome of Arthroscopic Anterior Cruciate Ligament Repair of Proximal Tears Using Knotless Single Suture Anchor Technique [32]

This is a machine-generated summary of:

Chitten, Jojin Jose; Arora, Manit: A Prospective Observational Study on Short-Term Functional Outcome of Arthroscopic Anterior Cruciate Ligament Repair of Proximal Tears Using Knotless Single Suture Anchor Technique [32]

Published in: Indian Journal of Orthopaedics (2021)

Link to original: https://doi.org/10.1007/s43465-021-00487-2

If you want to cite the papers, please refer to the original.

For technical reasons we could not place the page where the original quote is coming from.

Research Highlights

Anterior cruciate ligament (ACL) injuries are a common and debilitating issue, accounting for a significant percentage of knee ligament injuries and leading to considerable morbidity. While arthroscopic ACL reconstruction has been the standard treatment since 1980s and early 1990s, it is not without drawbacks, such as graft morbidity and failure to fully restore joint kinematics. Chitten et al. addresses these concerns by investigating the short-term functional outcomes of arthroscopic primary ACL repair using a single anchor surgical technique.

This prospective observational study was conducted at a tertiary care hospital with rigorous patient selection criteria. The research included patients who underwent arthroscopic primary ACL repair between specific years, with follow-ups at intervals up to 6 months. All surgeries were performed by a single experienced surgeon, and patient consent was obtained after thorough preoperative assessment. The inclusion criteria focused on proximal ACL tears with good tissue quality, while exclusion criteria ruled out cases such as delayed tears or poor tissue quality.

The surgical technique involved minimal bone work and aimed to preserve the native ligament to potentially improve joint kinematics and reduce recovery time. Post-operative protocols were standardized across patients, with regular clinical assessments and functional outcome measures taken using validated instruments like the IKDC and Lysholm score.

The key findings from this study indicate that arthroscopic primary ACL repair can lead to excellent short-term outcomes in carefully selected patients. A significant percentage of participants achieved clinically stable knees at 6 months post-operation, with marked improvements in pain relief and functional scores early in the post-operative period. These results suggest that primary ACL repair could be a viable alternative to reconstruction in specific cases, potentially offering faster rehabilitation and less morbidity associated with graft harvesting.

The results point towards an interesting concept of a 'yield point' at 6 weeks post-surgery, where maximal recovery is observed, which could guide clinicians in predicting long-term outcomes. However, as the authors note, further research is needed to validate this yield point and to assess long-term results beyond the 6-month follow-up.

This study contributes valuable insights into the potential benefits of arthroscopic primary ACL repair with single anchor technique for proximal tears. It opens up avenues for future research on patient selection criteria, long-term outcomes, and cost-effectiveness compared to traditional reconstruction methods.

In-Office Needle Arthroscopic Assessment after Primary ACL Repair: Short-Term Results in 15 Patients [33]

This is a machine-generated summary of:

Annibaldi, Alessandro; Monaco, Edoardo; Daggett, Matthew; Carrozzo, Alessandro; Mazza, Daniele; Previ, Leonardo; Rossi, Giorgio; Orlandi, Pierfrancesco; Ferretti, Andrea: In-office needle arthroscopic assessment after primary ACL repair: short-term results in 15 patients [33]

Published in: Journal of Experimental Orthopaedics (2022)

Link to original: https://doi.org/10.1186/s40634-022-00528-1

If you want to cite the papers, please refer to the original.

For technical reasons we could not place the page where the original quote is coming from.

Research Highlights

The evolution of arthroscopic surgery and orthopedic devices has rekindled interest in the primary repair of anterior cruciate ligament (ACL) injuries, particularly for proximal tears. Despite the historical shift from primary ACL repair to ACL reconstruction (ACLR) due to concerns over long-term stability and pain, recent studies suggest that primary repair may yield favorable outcomes. Annibaldi et al. aims to evaluate the efficacy of in-office needle arthroscopy as a diagnostic tool for assessing the healing of repaired ACLs compared to magnetic resonance imaging (MRI).

Annibaldi conducted a prospective study on patients with acute ACL tears, selecting those suitable for repair based on lesion type and tissue quality. The repaired ACLs were examined using in-office needle arthroscopy at an average follow-up of 7.2 months post-operation, prior to patients returning to sports activities. This minimally invasive technique involved local anesthesia, sterile saline injection for joint distension, and the use of a Nanoscope for direct visualization and probing of the ligament. The study also included MRI assessments and clinical evaluations using established scoring systems such as the Tegner Lysholm Knee Scoring Scale and the Knee Injury and Osteoarthritis Outcome Score.

The findings indicate that in-office needle arthroscopy is not only safe, but also provides reliable insights into the healing status of repaired ACLs. The technique allowed for direct assessment of ligament continuity, tension, and synovial coverage, with results showing significant correlations with MRI findings and biomechanical properties measured by KT-1000 arthrometry. These promising results suggest that primary ACL repair could be a viable alternative to ACLR for certain patient populations, provided accurate patient selection criteria are met.

This research supports the use of in-office needle arthroscopy as an effective diagnostic tool for evaluating repaired ACLs. This approach offers a cost-effective alternative to MRI with immediate post-procedure recovery, potentially influencing future diagnostic protocols and treatment strategies for ACL injuries.

Bibliography

1. Robson A. Ruptured cruciate ligaments and their repair by operation. Ann Surg. 1903;37(5):716–8.
2. Warren RF. Primary repair of the anterior cruciate ligament. Clin Orthop Relat Res. 1983;172:65–70.
3. Marshall JL, Warren RF, Wickiewicz TL. Primary surgical treatment of anterior cruciate ligament lesions. Am J Sports Med. 1982;10(2):103–7.
4. Sherman MF, Bonamo JR. Primary repair of the anterior cruciate ligament. Clin Sports Med. 1988;7(4):739–50.
5. Sherman MF, Lieber L, Bonamo JR, Podesta L, Reiter I. The long-term followup of primary anterior cruciate ligament repair. Defining a rationale for augmentation. Am J Sports Med. 1991;19(3):243–55.
6. DiFelice GS, Villegas C, Taylor S. Anterior cruciate ligament preservation: early results of a novel arthroscopic technique for suture anchor primary anterior cruciate ligament repair. Arthroscopy. 2015;31(11):2162–71.
7. Tibor L, Chan PH, Funahashi TT, Wyatt R, Maletis GB, Inacio MCS. Surgical technique trends in primary ACL reconstruction from 2007 to 2014. J Bone Joint Surg Am. 2016;98(13):1079–89.

8. Samuelsen BT, Webster KE, Johnson NR, Hewett TE, Krych AJ. Hamstring autograft versus patellar tendon autograft for ACL reconstruction: is there a difference in graft failure rate? A meta-analysis of 47,613 patients. Clin Orthop Relat Res. 2017;475(10):2459–68.
9. Gabler CM, Jacobs CA, Howard JS, Mattacola CG, Johnson DL. Comparison of graft failure rate between autografts placed via an anatomic anterior cruciate ligament reconstruction technique: a systematic review, meta-analysis, and meta-regression. Am J Sports Med. 2016;44(4):1069–79.
10. Irarrázaval S, Kurosaka M, Cohen M, Fu FH. Anterior cruciate ligament reconstruction. J ISAKOS Jt Disord Orthop Sport Med. 2016;1(1):38–52.
11. van Eck CF, Lesniak BP, Schreiber VM, Fu FH. Anatomic single- and double-bundle anterior cruciate ligament reconstruction flowchart. Arthroscopy. 2010;26(2):258–68.
12. Wright RW, Gill CS, Chen L, et al. Outcome of revision anterior cruciate ligament reconstruction: a systematic review. J Bone Joint Surg Am. 2012;94(6):531–6.
13. Andriolo L, Filardo G, Kon E, et al. Revision anterior cruciate ligament reconstruction: clinical outcome and evidence for return to sport. Knee Surg Sport Traumatol Arthrosc. 2015;23(10):2825–45.
14. Grassi A, Ardern CL, Muccioli G, Neri MP, Marcacci M, Zaffagnini S. Does revision ACL reconstruction measure up to primary surgery ? A meta-analysis comparing outcomes and radiographic results. Br J Sports Med. 2016;50:716–24.
15. van der List JP, DiFelice GS. Range of motion and complications following primary repair versus reconstruction of the anterior cruciate ligament. Knee. 2017;24(4):798–807.
16. van der List JP, DiFelice GS. Preoperative magnetic resonance imaging predicts eligibility for arthroscopic primary anterior cruciate ligament repair. Knee Surg Sport Traumatol Arthrosc. 2018;26:660. https://doi.org/10.1007/s00167-017-4646-z.
17. Bencardino JT, Beltran J, Feldman MI, Rose DJ. MR imaging of complications of anterior cruciate ligament graft reconstruction. Radiographics. 2009;29(7):2115–26.
18. Casagranda BC, Maxwell NJ, Kavanagh EC, Towers JD, Shen W, Fu FH. Normal appearance and complications of double-bundle and selective-bundle anterior cruciate ligament reconstructions using optimal MRI techniques. Am J Roentgenol. 2009;192(5):1407–15.
19. Meyers AB, Haims AH, Menn K, Moukaddam H. Imaging of anterior cruciate ligament repair and its complications. Am J Roentgenol. 2010;194(2):476–84.
20. Claes S, Verdonk P, Forsyth R, Bellemans J. The "ligamentization" process in anterior cruciate ligament reconstruction: what happens to the human graft? A systematic review of the literature. Am J Sports Med. 2011;39(11):2476–83.
21. Pauzenberger L, Syré S, Schurz M. "Ligamentization" in hamstring tendon grafts after anterior cruciate ligament reconstruction: a systematic review of the literature and a glimpse into the future. Arthroscopy. 2013;29(10):1712–21.
22. Hirschmann MT, Muller W. Complex function of the knee joint: the current understanding of the knee. Knee Surg Sports Traumatology Arthroscopy. 2015;23:2780–8.
23. van der List JP, DiFelice GS. Role of tear location on outcomes of open primary repair of the anterior cruciate ligament: a systematic review of historical studies. Knee. 2017;24(898–908):47.
24. van Eck CF, Limpisvasti O, ElAttrache NS. Is there a role for internal bracing and repair of the anterior cruciate ligament? A systematic literature review. Am J Sports Med. 2017;46:2291–8.
25. Achtnich A, Herbst E, Forkel P, et al. Acute proximal anterior cruciate ligament tears: outcomes after arthroscopic suture anchor repair versus anatomic single-bundle reconstruction. Arthroscopy. 2016;32:2562–9.
26. Hoffmann C, et al. Primary single suture anchor re-fixation of anterior cruciate ligament proximal avulsion tears leads to good functional mid-term results: a preliminary study in 12 patients. J Orthop Surg Res. 2017;12:17.
27. Ahn JH, Yoo JC, Yang HS, Kim JH, Wang JH. Second- look arthroscopic findings of 208 patients after ACL reconstruction. Knee Surg Sports Traumatol Arthrosc. 2007;15:242–8.

28. Mae T, Shino K, Nakagawa S. Second-look arthroscopy after anatomic anterior cruciate ligament reconstruction: bone- patellar tendon-bone versus hamstring tendon graft. J Orthop Sci. 2019;24:488–93.
29. Voigt JD, Mosier M, Huber B. Diagnostic needle arthroscopy and the economics of improved diagnostic accuracy: a cost analysis. Appl Health Econ Health Policy. 2014;12:523–35.
30. Zhang K, Crum RJ, Samuelsson K, Cadet E, Ayeni OR, de Sa D. In-office needle arthroscopy: a systematic review of indications and clinical utility. Arthroscopy. 2019;35:2709–21.
31. Daniels SP, van der List JP, Kazam JJ, DiFelice GS. Arthroscopic primary repair of the anterior cruciate ligament: what the radiologist needs to know. Skeletal Radiol. 2017;47:619. https://doi.org/10.1007/s00256-017-2857-5.
32. Chitten JJ, Arora M. A prospective observational study on short-term functional outcome of arthroscopic anterior cruciate ligament repair of proximal tears using knotless single suture anchor technique. Indian J Orthop. 2021;56:437. https://doi.org/10.1007/s43465-021-00487-2.
33. Annibaldi A, Monaco E, Daggett M, Carrozzo A, Mazza D, Previ L, Rossi G, Orlandi P, Ferretti A. In-office needle arthroscopic assessment after primary ACL repair: short-term results in 15 patients. J Exp Orthop. 2022;9:289. https://doi.org/10.1186/s40634-022-00528-1.

Chapter 11
Autograft Reconstruction

Alfred J. Tria Jr. and Giles R. Scuderi

Machine generated keywords: tunnel, muscle strength, network, muscle, angle, sagittal, graft angle, people, position, bayesian, old, bayesian network, network meta-analysis, healthy, healthy knee

Long-Term Results After Anterior Cruciate Ligament Reconstruction Using Patellar Tendon Versus Hamstring Tendon Autograft with a Minimum Follow-Up of 10 Years—A Systematic Review [44]

This is a machine-generated summary of:

Sollberger, V. D.; Korthaus, A.; Barg, A.; Pagenstert, G.: Long-term results after anterior cruciate ligament reconstruction using patellar tendon versus hamstring tendon autograft with a minimum follow-up of 10 years—a systematic review [44]

Published in: Archives of Orthopaedic and Trauma Surgery (2022)

Link to original: https://doi.org/10.1007/s00402-022-04687-9

A. J. Tria Jr. (✉)
Department of Orthopedics, Rutgers-Robert Wood Johnson Medical School, New Brunswick, NJ, USA

G. R. Scuderi
Northwell Health Orthopaedic Institute, New York, NY, USA

A. J. Tria Jr., G. R. Scuderi (eds.), *Ligaments of the Knee*,
https://doi.org/10.1007/978-3-031-66615-5_11

If you want to cite the papers, please refer to the original.

For technical reasons we could not place the page where the original quote is coming from.

Research Highlights

Anterior cruciate ligament (ACL) injuries are prevalent, particularly among younger individuals, and can lead to osteoarthritis (OA) years post-reconstruction. Despite various graft options for ACL reconstruction, the optimal choice remains contentious. Sollberger et al. seeks to elucidate long-term outcomes comparing bone-patellar tendon-bone (BPTB) and hamstring tendon (HT) autografts, focusing on patient-oriented outcomes, radiographic evidence of OA, and clinical stability.

This systematic review adheres to PRISMA guidelines and excludes studies with less than ten years of follow-up or those not meeting rigorous inclusion criteria. The review extracts data from nine eligible studies, encompassing patient-reported outcomes, clinical tests, and radiographic OA assessments. The authors note a shift in graft preference over time, with BPTB usage declining due to donor site morbidity concerns despite its association with lower revision rates in Scandinavian registry studies. The methodology includes independent data extraction by two authors and quality assessment using a modified Coleman Methodology Score.

The research highlights nuanced findings: no significant superiority of either graft type in long-term patient outcomes or graft rupture rates, but trends suggest BPTB may offer better stability and activity levels at the cost of higher donor site morbidity and OA incidence. HT grafts appear to have less donor site morbidity and better KOOS and IKDC-SKF scores. These insights are pivotal for individualized graft selection, considering factors like occupation or sports participation levels. Future research should include more long-term studies and consider the quadriceps tendon as another graft option, given its emerging relevance in ACL reconstruction.

Quadriceps Tendon Autograft for Primary ACL Reconstruction: A Bayesian Network Meta-analysis [45]

This is a machine-generated summary of:

Migliorini, Filippo; Eschweiler, Jörg; Mansy, Yasser El; Quack, Valentin; Tingart, Markus; Driessen, Arne: Quadriceps tendon autograft for primary ACL reconstruction: a Bayesian network meta-analysis [45]

Published in: European Journal of Orthopaedic Surgery & Traumatology (2020)
Link to original: https://doi.org/10.1007/s00590-020-02680-9

If you want to cite the papers, please refer to the original.

For technical reasons we could not place the page where the original quote is coming from.

Research Highlights

The anterior cruciate ligament (ACL) is crucial for knee stability, and its rupture is a common injury among active individuals, with an estimated 100,000 to 200,000 cases annually in the USA. If left unrepaired, a torn ACL can lead to joint instability and further degeneration, making surgical reconstruction necessary. While patellar tendon (PT) autografts are often considered the best option for ACL reconstruction, the quadriceps tendon (QT) autograft has recently gained attention for potentially superior outcomes. Migliorini et al. reviewed the efficacy of QT autografts compared to PT and hamstring tendon (HT) autografts through a Bayesian network meta-analysis.

The study involved a comprehensive literature search across multiple databases, adhering to PRISMA guidelines. Studies were selected based on stringent criteria, ensuring high-quality evidence by including only those with level I to III evidence and quantitative data on specific outcomes. The aim was to provide a robust comparison between QT and traditional PT or HT autografts.The analysis incorporated data from knees with a mean follow-up of 35 months, comparing clinical scores, joint stability measures, and post-operative complications. The statistical approach used a Bayesian hierarchical random-effect model and various tests to ensure the reliability of their findings.

The key findings suggest that QT autografts may be a viable alternative for primary ACL reconstruction, showing lower failure rates compared to PT and HT grafts and reduced anterior knee pain when compared to PT grafts. Clinical scores and joint laxity assessments indicated comparable outcomes among the different graft types. The results support the consideration of QT autografts not only for revision surgeries but also as a primary option.. However, the authors acknowledge limitations such as the preliminary nature of QT procedures and call for further research to strengthen evidence.

Graft Position in Arthroscopic Anterior Cruciate Ligament Reconstruction: Anteromedial Versus Transtibial Technique [46]

This is a machine-generated summary of:

Guler, Olcay; Mahırogulları, Mahir; Mutlu, Serhat; Cercı, Mehmet H.; Seker, Ali; Cakmak, Selami: Graft position in arthroscopic anterior cruciate ligament reconstruction: anteromedial versus transtibial technique [46]

Published in: Archives of Orthopaedic and Trauma Surgery (2016)

Link to original: https://doi.org/10.1007/s00402-016-2532-7

If you want to cite the papers, please refer to the original.

For technical reasons we could not place the page where the original quote is coming from.

Research Highlights

The restoration of knee function following anterior cruciate ligament (ACL) reconstruction is highly dependent on the placement of the graft, with previous studies underscoring the importance of anatomical positioning. Despite advancements in surgical techniques, achieving a graft angle that replicates the natural ACL remains a challenge. Guler et al. delved into the comparison of ACL graft angles and tunnel positions in reconstructions performed using anteromedial (AM) and transtibial (TT) techniques, aiming to assess their outcomes against those of healthy knees.

This retrospective analysis encompassed 116 knees from patients who underwent arthroscopic ACL reconstruction with hamstring tendon grafts. The authors compared postoperative MRI scans to evaluate the orientation and placement of the grafts. They employed rigorous inclusion and exclusion criteria to ensure a homogeneous study population, with all procedures being conducted by two experienced surgeons specialized in either AM or TT techniques. The study design was further reinforced by blinding three orthopedic surgeons during MRI evaluations to eliminate bias. Statistical analyses were conducted to compare functional outcomes using established scoring systems, providing a comprehensive assessment of each technique's efficacy.

The study's main advance is the finding that the AM technique may offer superior anatomical graft positioning compared to the TT technique, despite both methods aiming for anatomical accuracy. The findings suggest that while neither technique perfectly replicates natural ACL angles on the sagittal plane, functional outcomes between AM and TT reconstructions do not significantly differ. This study sets the stage for subsequent investigations that could ultimately enhance ACL reconstruction techniques and patient outcomes.

Age-Related Differences in Hamstring Tendon Used as Autograft in Reconstructive Anterior Cruciate Ligament Surgery [47]

This is a machine-generated summary of:

Naot, Dorit; Choi, Ally J.; Street, Matthew; Pronk, Madison; Zhao, Alex; Thambyah, Ashvin; Gao, Ryan; Cornish, Jillian; Dalbeth, Nicola; Coleman, Brendan; Musson, David S.: Age-related differences in hamstring tendon used as autograft in reconstructive anterior cruciate ligament surgery [47]

Published in: International Orthopaedics (2022)

Link to original: https://doi.org/10.1007/s00264-021-05285-x

If you want to cite the papers, please refer to the original.

For technical reasons we could not place the page where the original quote is coming from.

Research Highlights

Tears of the anterior cruciate ligament (ACL) are significant injuries affecting young, active individuals, with a high incidence in the USA annually. While surgical reconstruction using autografts is common, particularly from the bone-patellar-tendon-bone and hamstring tendon, these procedures are not without complications. Naot et al. addresses the observed higher failure rates of hamstring tendon autografts in younger patients by investigating the intrinsic properties of these tendons across different age groups.

Patients undergoing primary ACL reconstruction with hamstring autografts were recruited, ensuring ethical compliance and informed consent. The authors collected tendon samples during surgery for comprehensive analysis, including electron microscopy for structural imaging and microarray analysis for gene expression profiling. Biomechanical properties were assessed through rigorous testing to determine Young's modulus—a measure of stiffness—among other parameters. The methodology aimed to uncover age-related differences in tendon properties that could influence surgical outcomes.

The findings reveal that hamstring tendons from younger patients exhibit a higher Young's modulus compared to older counterparts, suggesting increased stiffness that may predispose these grafts to higher failure rates post-ACL reconstruction. Despite similar collagen fibril diameters across age groups, gene expression analysis highlighted distinct profiles in younger tendons, including genes involved in cell adhesion and inflammation. These molecular insights pave the way for future research into how tendon properties influence graft performance and could inform tailored approaches to ACL reconstruction based on patient age.

In conclusion, this study advances our understanding of the biological factors contributing to ACL reconstruction success and highlights the need for age-specific strategies in orthopaedic surgery. As Naot et al. suggest, further exploration into the relationship between tendon stiffness, gene expression patterns, and clinical outcomes is essential to optimize treatment for ACL injuries across different age groups.

Revision Anterior Cruciate Ligament Reconstruction Using the Ipsilateral Quadriceps Tendon Autograft: A Modular Reconstructive Option [48]

This is a machine-generated summary of:

Abouheif, Mohamed; Sharaby, Mohamed M. F.: Revision anterior cruciate ligament reconstruction using the ipsilateral Quadriceps tendon autograft: a modular reconstructive option [48]

Published in: International Orthopaedics (2023)

Link to original: https://doi.org/10.1007/s00264-023-05878-8

If you want to cite the papers, please refer to the original.

For technical reasons we could not place the page where the original quote is coming from.

Research Highlights

Anterior cruciate ligament (ACL) reconstruction is a common orthopedic procedure, but failure of the reconstructed ACL can occur due to trauma or cumulative stresses, often exacerbated by mechanical or biological factors such as non-anatomical tunnel placement or failure of graft ligamentization. Revision surgery presents unique challenges, including the choice of graft substitute to minimize additional morbidity Abouheif et al. proposes the use of ipsilateral quadriceps tendon autograft in revision ACL surgery as a modular option that can be tailored to suit dilated tunnels, potentially reducing morbidity and improving functional outcomes.

Prospective clinical series included patients with failed primary ACL reconstructions initially treated with hamstring autografts. The study evaluated candidates for revision surgery, excluding those with complicating factors such as multiple revisions or additional ligament injuries. The authors employed CT scans and MRI to precisely tailor the quadriceps tendon autograft to the dilated tunnels encountered during revision surgery. The authors found that the ipsilateral quadriceps tendon autograft offers a customizable solution that addresses the complexities of revision ACL surgery. The authors included postoperative assessments using the International Knee Documentation Committee (IKDC) subjective and objective testing and KT-1000 arthrometer measurements to objectively assess anterior tibial translation.

This represents a significant advance in revision ACL surgery, demonstrating that ipsilateral quadriceps tendon autografts can be effectively adapted for individual patient anatomy, leading to satisfactory functional outcomes with minimal morbidity. The authors concluded that the quadriceps tendon is not only versatile but also reliable for revision ACL reconstruction. Looking forward, this research opens avenues for further comparative studies on graft options in revision surgeries and underscores the importance of personalized surgical planning based on detailed preoperative assessments.

Anterior Cruciate Ligament Reconstruction Using Quadriceps Tendon Autograft Is a Viable Option for Small-Statured Female Patients [49]

This is a machine-generated summary of:

Goto, Kazumi; Duthon, Victoria B.; Menetrey, Jacques: Anterior cruciate ligament reconstruction using quadriceps tendon autograft is a viable option for small-statured female patients [49]

Published in: Knee Surgery, Sports Traumatology, Arthroscopy (2022)

Link to original: https://doi.org/10.1007/s00167-021-06845-9

If you want to cite the papers, please refer to the original.

For technical reasons we could not place the page where the original quote is coming from.

Research Highlights

Anterior cruciate ligament (ACL) injuries are a prevalent concern among athletes, often necessitating surgical intervention through ACL reconstruction. The selection of an appropriate graft—whether quadriceps tendon (QT), bone-patellar tendon-bone (BPTB), or hamstring tendon (HT)—remains a subject of debate, with recent literature suggesting the QT autograft as a promising candidate. Despite its reported advantages, including less harvest site pain and comparable clinical outcomes, the suitability of QT autografts for individuals of smaller stature, particularly in Asian countries, has been questioned due to potential complications such as donor site morbidity or loss of muscle strength. Goto et al. addresses this by comparing post-operative muscle strength and morbidity following ACL reconstruction with QT autografts across different patient statures.

This study involved female patients who underwent primary ACL reconstruction using QT autografts, excluding those with prior knee trauma or surgery, muscle injuries, or comorbidities affecting lower limb strength. Patients were divided into two groups based on height to assess the impact of stature on postoperative outcomes. The study followed standardized surgical techniques and postoperative protocols to ensure consistency across cases. Muscle strength was evaluated using an isokinetic dynamometer, and readiness to return to sports was assessed through the ACL-return to sport after injury scale.

The findings are significant: no notable differences were observed in muscle strength recovery or donor site morbidity between small- and large-statured patients post-ACL reconstruction with QT autografts. These results suggest that concerns over using QT grafts in smaller-statured individuals may be unfounded, providing reassurance for surgeons operating within diverse populations. The authors noted that the results support the notion that QT autografts for small-statured patients is a viable option without the risk of significant postoperative muscle weakness, marking a step forward in personalized ACL reconstruction strategies.

Bibliography

1. Coleman BD, Khan KM, Maffulli N, Cook JL, Wark JD. Studies of surgical outcome after patellar tendinopathy: clinical significance of methodological deficiencies and guidelines for future studies. Victorian Institute of Sport Tendon Study Group. Scand J Med Sci Sports. 2000;10:2–11.
2. Arnold MP, Calcei JG, Vogel N, Magnussen RA, Clatworthy M, Spalding T, et al. ACL Study Group survey reveals the evolution of anterior cruciate ligament reconstruction graft choice over the past three decades. Knee Surg Sports Traumatol Arthrosc. 2021;29:3871–6.
3. Keays SL, Newcombe PA, Bullock-Saxton JE, Bullock MI, Keays AC. Factors involved in the development of osteoarthritis after anterior cruciate ligament surgery. Am J Sports Med. 2010;38:455–63.
4. Mohtadi NG, Chan DS, Dainty KN, Whelan DB. Patellar tendon versus hamstring tendon autograft for anterior cruciate ligament rupture in adults. Cochrane Database Syst Rev. 2011;2011:CD005960. https://doi.org/10.1002/14651858.CD005960.pub2CD005960.
5. Keays SL, Bullock-Saxton JE, Keays AC, Newcombe PA, Bullock MI. A 6-year follow-up of the effect of graft site on strength, stability, range of motion, function, and joint degeneration after anterior cruciate ligament reconstruction: patellar tendon versus semitendinosus and Gracilis tendon graft. Am J Sports Med. 2007;35:729–39.
6. Pinczewski LA, Lyman J, Salmon LJ, Russell VJ, Roe J, Linklater J. A 10-year comparison of anterior cruciate ligament reconstructions with hamstring tendon and patellar tendon autograft: a controlled, prospective trial. Am J Sports Med. 2007;35:564–74.
7. Roe J, Pinczewski LA, Russell VJ, Salmon LJ, Kawamata T, Chew M. A 7-year follow-up of patellar tendon and hamstring tendon grafts for arthroscopic anterior cruciate ligament reconstruction: differences and similarities. Am J Sports Med. 2005;33:1337–45.

8. Lecoq FA, Parienti JJ, Murison J, Ruiz N, Bouacida K, Besse J, et al. Graft choice and the incidence of osteoarthritis after anterior cruciate ligament reconstruction: a causal analysis from a cohort of 541 patients. Am J Sports Med. 2018;46:2842–50.
9. Bjornsson H, Samuelsson K, Sundemo D, Desai N, Sernert N, Rostgard-Christensen L, et al. A randomized controlled trial with mean 16-year follow-up comparing hamstring and patellar tendon autografts in anterior cruciate ligament reconstruction. Am J Sports Med. 2016;44:2304–13.
10. Thompson SM, Salmon LJ, Waller A, Linklater J, Roe JP, Pinczewski LA. Twenty-year outcome of a longitudinal prospective evaluation of isolated endoscopic anterior cruciate ligament reconstruction with patellar tendon or hamstring autograft. Am J Sports Med. 2016;44:3083–94.
11. Sajovic M, Stropnik D, Skaza K. Long-term comparison of semitendinosus and gracilis tendon versus patellar tendon autografts for anterior cruciate ligament reconstruction: a 17-year follow-up of a randomized controlled trial. Am J Sports Med. 2018;46:1800–8.
12. Harris NL, Smith D, Lamoreaux L, Purnell M. Central quadriceps tendon for anterior cruciate ligament reconstruction. Part I: morphometric and biomechanical evaluation. Am J Sports Med. 1997;25:23–8.
13. Stäubli HU, Schatzmann L, Brunner P, Rincón L, Nolte LP. Quadriceps tendon and patellar ligament: cryosectional anatomy and structural properties in young adults. Knee Surg Sports Traumatol Arthrosc. 1996;4:100–10.
14. Reinhardt KR, Hetsroni I, Marx RG. Graft selection for anterior cruciate ligament reconstruction: a level I systematic review comparing failure rates and functional outcomes. Orthop Clin North Am. 2010;41(2):249–62. https://doi.org/10.1016/j.ocl.2009.12.009.
15. Hantes ME, Zachos VC, Liantsis A, Venouziou A, Karantanas AH, Malizos KN. Differences in graft orientation using the transtibial and anteromedial portal technique in anterior cruciate ligament reconstruction: a magnetic resonance imaging study. Knee Surg Sports Traumatol Arthrosc. 2009;17:880–6.
16. Ahn JH, Lee SH, Yoo JC, Ha HC. Measurement of the graft angles for the anterior cruciate ligament reconstruction with transtibial technique using postoperative magnetic resonance imaging in comparative study. Knee Surg Sports Traumatol Arthrosc. 2007;15:1293–300.
17. Cho Y, Cho J, Kim D. Normal sagittal of the anterior cruciate ligament can be reproduced using accessory anteromedial portal technique: a magnetic resonance imaging study. Arch Orthop Trauma Surg. 2012;132:1011–9.
18. Rayan F, Nanjayan SK, Quah C, Ramoutar D, Konan S, Haddad FS. Review of evolution of tunnel position in anterior cruciate ligament reconstruction. World J Orthop. 2015;6:252–62.
19. Tegner Y, Lysholm J. Rating systems in the evaluation of knee ligament injuries. Clin Orthop Relat Res. 1985;198:43–9.
20. Bowers AL, Bedi A, Lipman JD, Potter HG, Rodeo SA, Pearle AD, Warren RF, Altchek DW. Comparison of anterior cruciate ligament tunnel position and graft obliquity with transtibial and anteromedial portal femoral tunnel reaming techniques using high-resolution magnetic resonance imaging. Arthroscopy. 2011;27:1511–22.
21. Marchant BG, Noyes FR, Barber-Westin SD, Fleckenstein C. Prevalence of nonanatomical graft placement in a series of failed anterior cruciate ligament reconstructions. Am J Sports Med. 2010;38:1987–96.
22. DeFazio MW, Curry EJ, Gustin MJ, Sing DC, Abdul-Rassoul H, Ma R, Fu F, Li X. Return to sport after ACL reconstruction with a BTB versus hamstring tendon autograft: a systematic review and meta-analysis. Orthop J Sports Med. 2020;8:2325967120964919. https://doi.org/10.1177/2325967120964919.
23. Rahardja R, Zhu M, Love H, Clatworthy MG, Monk AP, Young SW. Factors associated with revision following anterior cruciate ligament reconstruction: a systematic review of registry data. Knee. 2020;27:287–99. https://doi.org/10.1016/j.knee.2019.12.003.

24. Jelinsky SA, Archambault J, Li L, Seeherman H. Tendon-selective genes identified from rat and human musculoskeletal tissues. J Orthop Res. 2010;28:289–97. https://doi.org/10.1002/jor.20999.
25. Todor A, Caterev S, Nistor DV, Khallouki Y. Free bone plug quadriceps tendon harvest and suspensory button attachment for anterior cruciate ligament reconstruction. Arthrosc Tech. 2016;5:e541–4. https://doi.org/10.1016/j.eats.2016.02.001.
26. Xerogeanes JW. Quadriceps tendon graft for anterior cruciate ligament reconstruction: the graft of the future! Arthrosc: J Arthrosc Relat Surg: Off Publ Arthrosc Assoc N Ame Int Arthrosc Assoc. 2019;35:696–7. https://doi.org/10.1016/j.arthro.2019.01.011.
27. van Eck CF, Schreiber VM, Mejia HA, Samuelsson K, van Dijk CN, Karlsson J, Fu FH. "Anatomic" anterior cruciate ligament reconstruction: a systematic review of surgical techniques and reporting of surgical data. Arthroscopy. 2010;26(9 Suppl):S2–12.
28. Middleton KK, Hamilton T, Irrgang JJ, Karlsson J, Harner CD, Fu FH. Anatomic anterior cruciate ligament (ACL) reconstruction: a global perspective. Part 1. Knee Surg Sports Traumatol Arthrosc. 2014;22(7):1467–82.
29. Hadjicostas PT, Soucacos PN, Berger I, Koleganova N, Paessler HH. Comparative analysis of the morphologic structure of quadriceps and patellar tendon: a descriptive laboratory study. Arthroscopy. 2007;23:744–50.
30. Adams DJ, Mazzocca AD, Fulkerson JP. Residual strength of the quadriceps versus patellar tendon after harvesting a central free tendon graft. Arthroscopy. 2006;22:76–9.
31. Shani RH, Umpierez E, Nasert M. Biomechanical comparison of quadriceps and patellar tendon grafts in anterior cruciate ligament reconstruction. Arthroscopy. 2016;32(1):71–5.
32. Stäubli HU, Schatzmann L, Brunner P. Mechanical tensile properties of the quadriceps tendon and patellar ligament in young adults. Am J Sports Med. 1999;27(1):27–34.
33. Belk JW, Kraeutler MJ, Marshall HA, Goodrich JA, McCarty EC. Quadriceps tendon autograft for primary anterior cruciate ligament reconstruction: a systematic review of comparative studies with minimum 2-year follow-up. Arthroscopy. 2018;34:1699–707.
34. Gagliardi AG, Carry PM, Parikh HB, Albright JC. Outcomes of quadriceps tendon with patellar bone block anterior cruciate ligament reconstruction in adolescent patients with a minimum 2-year follow-up. Am J Sports Med. 2020;48(1):93–8.
35. Kim SJ, Kumar P, Oh KS. Anterior cruciate ligament reconstruction: autogenous quadriceps tendon-bone compared with bone-patellar tendon-bone grafts at 2-year follow-up. Arthroscopy. 2009;25(2):137–44. https://doi.org/10.1016/j.arthro.2008.09.014.
36. Lee JK, Lee S, Lee MC. Outcomes of anatomic anterior cruciate ligament reconstruction: bone-quadriceps tendon graft versus double-bundle hamstring tendon graft. Am J Sports Med. 2016;44(9):2323–9. https://doi.org/10.1177/0363546516650666.
37. Mouarbes D, Menetrey J, Vincent Marot V, Courtot L, Berard E, Cavaignac E. Anterior cruciate ligament reconstruction. A systematic review and meta-analysis of outcomes for quadriceps tendon autograft versus bone–patellar tendon–bone and hamstring-tendon autografts. Am J Sports Med. 2019;47(14):3531–40.
38. Nyland J, Collis P, Huffstutler A, Sachdeva S, Spears JR, Greene J, Caborn DNM. Quadriceps tendon autograft ACL reconstruction has less pivot shift laxity and lower failure rates than hamstring tendon autografts. Knee Surg Sports Traumatol Arthrosc. 2020;28(2):509–18.
39. Runer A, Csapo R, Hepperger C, Herbort M, Hoser C, Fink C. Anterior cruciate ligament reconstructions with quadriceps tendon autograft result in lower graft rupture rates but similar patient-reported outcomes as compared with hamstring tendon autograft: a comparison of 875 patients. Am J Sports Med. 2020;48(9):2195–204.
40. Andersson D, Samuelsson K, Karlsson J. Treatment of anterior cruciate ligament injuries with special reference to surgical technique and rehabilitation: an assessment of randomized controlled trials. Arthroscopy. 2009;25:653–85.
41. Johnston PT, Feller JA, McClelland JA, Webster KE. Knee strength deficits following anterior cruciate ligament reconstruction differ between quadriceps and hamstring tendon autografts. J ISAKOS. 2021;6(2):88–93. https://doi.org/10.1007/s00167-021-06565-0.

42. Cavaignac E, Coulin B, Tscholl P, Nik Mohd Fatmy N, Duthon V, Menetrey J. Is quadriceps tendon autograft a better choice than hamstring autograft for anterior cruciate ligament reconstruction? A comparative study with a mean follow-up of 3.6 years. Am J Sports Med. 2017;45(6):1326–32. https://doi.org/10.1177/0363546516688665.
43. Hunnicutt JL, Gregory CM, McLeod MM, Woolf SK, Chapin RW, Slone HS. Quadriceps recovery after anterior cruciate ligament reconstruction with quadriceps tendon versus patellar tendon autografts. Orthop J Sports Med. 2019;7(4):2325967119839786.
44. Sollberger VD, Korthaus A, Barg A, Pagenstert G. Long-term results after anterior cruciate ligament reconstruction using patellar tendon versus hamstring tendon autograft with a minimum follow-up of 10 years—a systematic review. Arch Orthop Trauma Surg. 2022;143:4277–89. https://doi.org/10.1007/s00402-022-04687-9.
45. Migliorini F, Eschweiler J, El Mansy Y, Quack V, Tingart M, Driessen A. Quadriceps tendon autograft for primary ACL reconstruction: a Bayesian network meta-analysis. Eur J Orthop Surg Traumatol. 2020;30:1129–38. https://doi.org/10.1007/s00590-020-02680-9.
46. Guler O, Mahırogulları M, Mutlu S, Cercı MH, Seker A, Cakmak S. Graft position in arthroscopic anterior cruciate ligament reconstruction: anteromedial versus transtibial technique. Arch Orthop Trauma Surg. 2016;136:1571–80. https://doi.org/10.1007/s00402-016-2532-7.
47. Naot D, Choi AJ, Street M, Pronk M, Zhao A, Thambyah A, Gao R, Cornish J, Dalbeth N, Coleman B, Musson DS. Age-related differences in hamstring tendon used as autograft in reconstructive anterior cruciate ligament surgery. Int Orthop. 2022;46:845–53. https://doi.org/10.1007/s00264-021-05285-x.
48. Abouheif M, Sharaby MMF. Revision anterior cruciate ligament reconstruction using the ipsilateral Quadriceps tendon autograft: a modular reconstructive option. Int Orthop. 2023;47:2967–76. https://doi.org/10.1007/s00264-023-05878-8.
49. Goto K, Duthon VB, Menetrey J. Anterior cruciate ligament reconstruction using quadriceps tendon autograft is a viable option for small-statured female patients. Knee Surg Sports Traumatol Arthrosc. 2022;30:2358–63. https://doi.org/10.1007/s00167-021-06845-9.

Chapter 12
Allograft Reconstruction

Alfred J. Tria Jr. and Giles R. Scuderi

Machine generated keywords: allograft, qtpb, group, stsb, stdb, qtpb allograft, reconstruction qtpb, qtpb autograft, stdb group, stsb group, group stdb, singletunnel, size, doublebundle, disease

Anterior Cruciate Ligament Reconstruction with Quadriceps Tendon-Patellar Bone Allograft: Matched Case Control Study [29]

This is a machine-generated summary of:

Kwak, Yoon-Ho; Lee, Sahnghoon; Lee, Myung Chul; Han, Hyuk-Soo: Anterior cruciate ligament reconstruction with quadriceps tendon-patellar bone allograft: matched case control study [29]

Published in: BMC Musculoskeletal Disorders (2018)

Link to original: https://doi.org/10.1186/s12891-018-1959-0

A. J. Tria Jr. (✉)
Department of Orthopedics, Rutgers-Robert Wood Johnson Medical School, New Brunswick, NJ, USA

G. R. Scuderi
Northwell Health Orthopaedic Institute, New York, NY, USA

A. J. Tria Jr., G. R. Scuderi (eds.), *Ligaments of the Knee*,
https://doi.org/10.1007/978-3-031-66615-5_12

If you want to cite the papers, please refer to the original.

For technical reasons we could not place the page where the original quote is coming from.

Research Highlights

Anterior cruciate ligament (ACL) reconstruction is a critical surgical procedure for restoring knee stability, with various graft options available. Despite the lower retear rates observed with autografts in younger individuals, the debate continues over the optimal graft choice. Kwak et al. evaluates clinical outcomes of ACL reconstruction using quadriceps tendon-patellar bone (QTPB) allografts versus autografts, focusing on knee stability, activity levels, and functional scores.

The retrospective study conducted at Seoul National University Hospital involved patients who underwent ACL reconstruction with QTPB grafts. The authors matched patients receiving allografts with those receiving autografts based on age and body mass index to ensure comparability. Preoperative and postoperative assessments included ligament laxity tests and functional scoring systems such as the International Knee Documentation Committee score and Knee Injury and Osteoarthritis Outcome Score. The QTPB allografts were sourced from Community Tissue Services, adhering to stringent testing standards to ensure safety and quality. The authors employed a modified transtibial technique for the surgical procedure, followed by a standardized rehabilitation protocol for all patients. Statistical analyses were performed using SPSS software, with significant findings determined at $P < 0.05$.

ACL reconstruction with QTPB allografts demonstrated comparable clinical outcomes to autografts in terms of knee stability and function at a follow-up of 31.2 months. The authors noted that the results suggest that QTPB allograft is a promising alternative for ACL reconstruction. While no reruptures were reported in the short-term follow-up, the authors acknowledge that long-term studies are necessary to fully assess outcomes, including rerupture rates.

Hamstring Tendon Autograft Versus Fresh-Frozen Tibialis Posterior Allograft in Primary Arthroscopic Anterior Cruciate Ligament Reconstruction: A Retrospective Cohort Study with Three to Six Years Follow-Up [30]

This is a machine-generated summary of:

Mardani-Kivi, Mohsen; Karimi-Mobarakeh, Mahmoud; Keyhani, Sohrab; Saheb-Ekhtiari, Khashayar; Hashemi-Motlagh, Keyvan; Sarvi, Ali: Hamstring tendon autograft versus fresh-frozen tibialis posterior allograft in primary arthroscopic anterior cruciate ligament reconstruction: a retrospective cohort study with three to six years follow-up [30]

Published in: International Orthopaedics (2016)

Link to original: https://doi.org/10.1007/s00264-016-3164-9

If you want to cite the papers, please refer to the original.

For technical reasons we could not place the page where the original quote is coming from.

Research Highlights

The anterior cruciate ligament (ACL) is crucial for knee stability, and its reconstruction is a common orthopedic procedure aimed at restoring function after injury. While hamstring tendon autografts (HT) have gained popularity due to improved fixation methods, allografts such as the tibialis posterior (TP) offer advantages like reduced donor site morbidity and surgery time. However, concerns about infection risk and long-term outcomes persist. Mardani-Kivi et al. addresses this by comparing the stability and function of knees after ACL reconstruction using single-loop TP allografts versus HT autografts.

This study was approved by the Local Ethical Committee of Guilan University of Medical Sciences, adhering to the Declaration of Helsinki. The research involved patients who underwent ACL reconstruction, with the surgeon favoring TP allografts for specific patient demographics. The study gathered demographic data, injury specifics, and both objective and subjective pre- and post-operative measures.

The surgical techniques employed were standardized across both groups, with non-irradiated fresh frozen TP grafts used for allografts and conventional harvesting methods for HT autografts. Post-operative care was consistent among participants, with follow-ups spanning 3 years to assess outcomes such as range of motion (ROM), side-to-side difference (SSD), and patient-reported satisfaction scores.

The study's findings reveal that both TP allografts and HT autografts provide satisfactory knee stability and function with similar post-operative complication rates. The results suggest that TP allografts are a viable option for ACL reconstruction, offering comparable outcomes to the more commonly used HT autografts.

Arthroscopic Reconstruction of Anterior Cruciate Ligaments with Allograft: Single-Tunnel Single-Bundle Versus Single-Tunnel Double-Bundle Techniques [31]

This is a machine-generated summary of:

Deng, Zhenhan; Zheng, Yizi; Deng, Zhiqin; Lu, Changwei; Wu, Yihua; Chen, Kang; Fu, Zicai; Zhang, Hui; Lu, Wei; Zhu, Weimin: Arthroscopic reconstruction of anterior cruciate ligaments with allograft: single-tunnel single-bundle versus single-tunnel double-bundle techniques [31]

Published in: Journal of Orthopaedics and Traumatology (2022)

Link to original: https://doi.org/10.1186/s10195-022-00649-4

If you want to cite the papers, please refer to the original.

For technical reasons we could not place the page where the original quote is coming from.

Research Highlights

The anterior cruciate ligament (ACL) is crucial for knee stability, with its anteromedial (AM) and posterolateral (PL) bundles each providing unique stabilizing functions. While single-tunnel single-bundle (STSB) ACL reconstructions are common, they may not fully restore rotational stability. Deng et al.addresses this issue by comparing the outcomes of STSB with single-tunnel double-bundle (STDB) reconstructions, hypothesizing that STDB could offer better knee stability without increasing complications.

The authors conducted a retrospective review of patients who underwent arthroscopic STSB or STDB ACL reconstruction with anterior tibialis tendon allografts. The inclusion criteria ensured patients had confirmed ACL ruptures and no significant osteochondral degeneration, while those with multiple ligament damage or partial ACL ruptures were excluded. All surgeries were performed by the same senior surgeon, and the allografts were prepared and implanted using meticulous techniques tailored to each reconstruction type. Postoperative care was standardized across both groups, and outcomes were measured using the International Knee Documentation Committee (IKDC), Lysholm, and Tegner scores, along with physical examinations.

The study's main advances include evidence that STDB reconstruction provides superior rotational stability compared to STSB without introducing additional complications. Deng et al. results showed significant improvements in knee function postoperatively in both groups, but the pivot shift test positive rate was significantly lower in the STDB group, indicating better rotational stability. Despite these promising findings, the authors acknowledge limitations such as the retrospective nature of the study and suggest that future research should include prospective randomized controlled trials to further validate their results. The comparison between STDB and double-tunnel double-bundle (DTDB) techniques also remains an area for future investigation.

Functional Results of Allograft vs. Autograft Tendons in Anterior Cruciate Ligament (ACL) Reconstruction at 10-Year Follow-Up [32]

This is a machine-generated summary of:

Bistolfi, Alessandro; Capella, Marcello; Guidotti, Claudio; Sabatini, Luigi; Artiaco, Stefano; Massè, Alessandro; Ferracini, Riccardo: Functional results of allograft vs. autograft tendons in anterior cruciate ligament (ACL) reconstruction at 10-year follow-up [32]

Published in: European Journal of Orthopaedic Surgery & Traumatology (2020)
Link to original: https://doi.org/10.1007/s00590-020-02823-y

If you want to cite the papers, please refer to the original.

For technical reasons we could not place the page where the original quote is coming from.

Research Highlights

Anterior cruciate ligament (ACL) tears are a prevalent injury, representing a significant percentage of all knee injuries, affecting not only professional athletes but also active individuals at various levels. The current standard for treating complete ACL tears is reconstruction surgery, which involves critical decisions regarding surgical techniques, such as the choice between autografts and allografts. Bistolfi et al. addresses the long-term effectiveness of allografts compared to autografts, focusing on clinical outcomes and complication rates over an extended follow-up period.

This study involved a meticulous selection process to compare patients who underwent ACL reconstruction with either allograft or autograft tissue at their institution. Their aim was to provide a clear comparison between the two techniques, considering long-term results.. The study enrolled patients who met specific inclusion criteria and were matched for age and gender. The allograft group consisted of patients with a minimum follow-up of 8 years, while the autograft group was selected to closely match this cohort. The surgical techniques for both groups were detailed, with particular attention to graft harvesting and positioning. Postoperative evaluations included physical examinations and scoring systems like the IKDC Questionnaire and Lysholm score to assess functional status.

This study presents significant findings that support the use of allografts as a viable option for ACL reconstruction in certain patient populations. The results indicate that allografts can provide comparable functional outcomes to autografts. With no major complications directly related to the allograft tissue reported, the research suggests that concerns over disease transmission and graft rejection may be mitigated with modern harvesting and sterilization techniques. While acknowledging limitations such as its retrospective nature and potential selection bias, the study contributes valuable insights into long-term patient outcomes post-ACL reconstruction. Looking forward, these findings could guide more personalized approaches to ACL surgery, particularly for middle-aged patients or those seeking to avoid donor-site morbidity without compromising their active lifestyles.

Bibliography

1. Geib TM, Shelton WR, Phelps RA, Clark L. Anterior cruciate ligament reconstruction using quadriceps tendon autograft: intermediate-term outcome. Arthroscopy. 2009;25(12):1408–14. https://doi.org/10.1016/j.arthro.2009.06.004.
2. Bottoni CR, Smith EL, Shaha J, Shaha SS, Raybin SG, Tokish JM, Rowles DJ. Autograft versus allograft anterior cruciate ligament reconstruction: a prospective, randomized clinical study with a minimum 10-year follow-up. Am J Sports Med. 2015;43:2501–9. https://doi.org/10.1177/0363546515596406.
3. Sun K, Tian S, Zhang J, Xia C, Zhang C, Yu T. Anterior cruciate ligament reconstruction with BPTB autograft, irradiated versus non-irradiated allograft: a prospective randomized clinical study. Knee Surg Sports Traumatol Arthrosc. 2009;17(5):464–74.
4. Lee JK, Lee S, Seong SC, Lee MC. Anatomic single-bundle ACL reconstruction is possible with use of the modified transtibial technique: a comparison with the anteromedial transportal technique. J Bone Joint Surg Am. 2014;96(8):664–72.
5. Gorschewsky O, Klakow A, Putz A, Mahn H, Neumann W. Clinical comparison of the autologous quadriceps tendon (BQT) and the autologous patella tendon (BPTB) for the reconstruction of the anterior cruciate ligament. Knee Surg Sports Traumatol Arthrosc. 2007;15(11):1284–92. https://doi.org/10.1007/s00167-007-0371-3.
6. Han HS, Seong SC, Lee S, Lee MC. Anterior cruciate ligament reconstruction : quadriceps versus patellar autograft. Clin Orthop Relat Res. 2008;466(1):198–204. https://doi.org/10.1007/s11999-007-0015-4.
7. Lee MC, Seong SC, Lee S, Chang CB, Park YK, Jo H, Kim CH. Vertical femoral tunnel placement results in rotational knee laxity after anterior cruciate ligament reconstruction. Arthroscopy. 2007;23(7):771–8.
8. Lee S, Seong SC, Jo H, Park YK, Lee MC. Outcome of anterior cruciate ligament reconstruction using quadriceps tendon autograft. Arthroscopy. 2004;20(8):795–802.
9. Lund B, Nielsen T, Fauno P, Christiansen SE, Lind M. Is quadriceps tendon a better graft choice than patellar tendon? A prospective randomized study. Arthroscopy. 2014;30(5):593–8. https://doi.org/10.1016/j.arthro.2014.01.012.
10. Kim SJ, Kumar P, Oh KS. Anterior cruciate ligament reconstruction: autogenous quadriceps tendon-bone compared with bone-patellar tendon-bone grafts at 2-year follow-up. Arthroscopy. 2009;25(2):137–44. https://doi.org/10.1016/j.arthro.2008.09.014.
11. Hu J, Qu J, Xu D, Zhou J, Lu H. Allograft versus autograft for anterior cruciate ligament reconstruction: an up-to-date meta-analysis of prospective studies. Int Orthop. 2013;37:311–20. https://doi.org/10.1007/s00264-012-1720-5.

12. Lawhorn KW, Howell SM, Traina SM, Gottlieb JE, Meade TD, Freedberg HI. The effect of graft tissue on anterior cruciate ligament outcomes: a multicenter, prospective, randomized controlled trial comparing autograft hamstrings with fresh-frozen anterior tibialis allograft. Arthroscopy. 2012;28:1079–86. https://doi.org/10.1016/j.arthro.2012.05.010.
13. Scheffler SU, Schmidt T, Gangey I, Dustmann M, Unterhauser F, Weiler A. Fresh-frozen free-tendon allografts versus autografts in anterior cruciate ligament reconstruction: delayed remodeling and inferior mechanical function during long-term healing in sheep. Arthroscopy. 2008;24:448–58. https://doi.org/10.1016/j.arthro.2007.10.011.
14. Pearsall Iv AW, Hollis JM, Russell GV Jr, Scheer Z. A biomechanical comparison of three lower extremity tendons for ligamentous reconstruction about the knee. Arthroscopy. 2003;19:1091–6. https://doi.org/10.1016/j.arthro.2003.10.1015.
15. Haut Donahue TL, Howell SM, Hull ML, Gregersen C. A biomechanical evaluation of anterior and posterior tibialis tendons as suitable single-loop anterior cruciate ligament grafts. Arthroscopy. 2002;18:589–97. https://doi.org/10.1053/jars.2002.32617.
16. Edgar CM, Zimmer S, Kakar S, Jones H, Schepsis AA. Prospective comparison of auto and allograft hamstring tendon constructs for ACL reconstruction. Clin Orthop Relat Res. 2008;466:2238–46. https://doi.org/10.1007/s11999-008-0305-5.
17. Nakata K, Shino K, Horibe S, Tanaka Y, Toritsuka Y, Nakamura N, Koyanagi M, Yoshikawa H. Arthroscopic anterior cruciate ligament reconstruction using fresh-frozen bone plug-free allogeneic tendons: 10-year follow-up. Arthroscopy. 2008;24:285–91. https://doi.org/10.1016/j.arthro.2007.09.007.
18. Zeng C, Gao SG, Li H, Yang T, Luo W, Li YS, Lei GH. Autografts versus allograft in anterior cruciate ligament reconstruction: a meta-analysis of randomized controlled trials and systematic review of overlapping systematic reviews. Arthroscopy. 2016;32:153–63. https://doi.org/10.1016/j.arthro.2015.07.027.
19. Ping LW, Bin S, Rui Y, Yang S, Zheng ZZ, Yue D. Arthroscopic ACL reconstruction with reverse "Y"-plasty grafts and fixation in the femur with either a bioabsorbable interference screw or an endobutton. Knee. 2012;19:78–83.
20. Li W, Song Y, Song B, Yang R, Xing T, Chen Z, et al. Comparison of anterior cruciate ligament reconstruction methods between reverse "Y" plasty reconstruction and traditional single-bundle technique—a cadaveric study. J Orthop Translat. 2018;14:1–7.
21. Debandi A, Maeyama A, Lu S, Hume C, Asai S, Goto B, et al. Biomechanical comparison of three anatomic ACL reconstructions in a porcine model. Knee Surg Sports Traumatol Arthrosc. 2011;19:728–35.
22. Barrett GR, Luber K, Replogle WH, Manley JL. Allograft anterior cruciate ligament reconstruction in the young, active patient: Tegner activity level and failure rate. Arthroscopy. 2010;26:1593–601.
23. Jackson DW, Grood ES, Goldstein JD, Rosen MA, Kurzweil PR, Cummings JF, Simon TM. A comparison of patellar tendon autograft and allograft used for anterior cruciate ligament reconstruction in the goat model. Am J Sports Med. 1993;21:176–85.
24. Malinin TI, Levitt RL, Bashore C, Temple HT, Mnaymneh W. A study of retrieved allografts used to replace anterior cruciate ligaments. Arthroscopy. 2002;18:163–70.
25. Shino K, Inoue M, Horibe S, Hamada M, Ono K. Reconstruction of the anterior cruciate ligament using allogeneic tendon. Long-term followup. Am J Sports Med. 1990;18(5):457–65.
26. Kaeding CC, Pedroza AD, Reinke EK, Huston LJ, Consortium M, Spindler KP. Risk factors and predictors of subsequent ACL injury in either knee after ACL reconstruction: prospective analysis of 2488 primary ACL reconstructions from the MOON cohort. Am J Sports Med. 2015;43(7):1583–90.
27. Padua R, Bondi R, Ceccarelli E, Bondi L, Romanini E, Zanoli G, et al. Italian version of the international knee documentation committee subjective knee form: cross-cultural adaptation and validation. Arthroscopy. 2004;20(8):819–23.

28. Cerciello S, Corona K, Morris BJ, Visonà E, Maccauro G, Maffulli N. Cross-cultural adaptation and validation of the Italian versions of the kujala, larsen, lysholm and fulkerson scores in patients with patellofemoral disorders. J OrthopTraumatol. 2018;19(1):18.
29. Kwak Y-H, Lee S, Lee MC, Han H-S. Anterior cruciate ligament reconstruction with quadriceps tendon-patellar bone allograft: matched case control study. BMC Musculoskelet Disord. 2018;19:45. https://doi.org/10.1186/s12891-018-1959-0.
30. Mardani-Kivi M, Karimi-Mobarakeh M, Keyhani S, Saheb-Ekhtiari K, Hashemi-Motlagh K, Sarvi A. Hamstring tendon autograft versus fresh-frozen tibialis posterior allograft in primary arthroscopic anterior cruciate ligament reconstruction: a retrospective cohort study with three to six years follow-up. Int Orthop. 2016;40:1905–11. https://doi.org/10.1007/s00264-016-3164-9.
31. Deng Z, Zheng Y, Deng Z, Lu C, Wu Y, Chen K, Fu Z, Zhang H, Lu W, Zhu W. Arthroscopic reconstruction of anterior cruciate ligaments with allograft: single-tunnel single-bundle versus single-tunnel double-bundle techniques. J Orthop Traumatol. 2022;23:26. https://doi.org/10.1186/s10195-022-00649-4.
32. Bistolfi A, Capella M, Guidotti C, Sabatini L, Artiaco S, Massè A, Ferracini R. Functional results of allograft vs. autograft tendons in anterior cruciate ligament (ACL) reconstruction at 10-year follow-up. Eur J Orthop Surg Traumatol. 2020;31:729–35. https://doi.org/10.1007/s00590-020-02823-y.

Chapter 13
Capsular Augmentations

Alfred J. Tria Jr. and Giles R. Scuderi

Machine generated keywords: augmentation, partial, bundle, partial acl, aclr, partial tear, symptomatic, oaaclr, overthetop, bundle augmentation, acl augmentation, lar augmentation, amateur athlete, professional amateur, fiber

Short Term Results of Anterior Cruciate Ligament Augmentation in Professional and Amateur Athletes [34]

This is a machine-generated summary of:

Yazdi, Hamidreza; Torkaman, Ali; Ghahramani, Morteza; Moradi, Amin; Nazarian, Ara; Ghorbanhoseini, Mohammad: Short term results of anterior cruciate ligament augmentation in professional and amateur athletes [34]

Published in: Journal of Orthopaedics and Traumatology (2017)

Link to original: https://doi.org/10.1007/s10195-017-0447-x

A. J. Tria Jr. (✉)
Department of Orthopedics, Rutgers-Robert Wood Johnson Medical School, New Brunswick, NJ, USA

G. R. Scuderi
Northwell Health Orthopaedic Institute, New York, NY, USA

A. J. Tria Jr., G. R. Scuderi (eds.), *Ligaments of the Knee*,
https://doi.org/10.1007/978-3-031-66615-5_13

If you want to cite the papers, please refer to the original.

For technical reasons we could not place the page where the original quote is coming from.

Research Highlights

Anterior cruciate ligament (ACL) injuries are a significant concern for athletes, with partial tears comprising a notable percentage of these injuries. Despite their prevalence, the epidemiology of partial ACL tears remains less understood than that of complete tears. Yazdi et al. evaluated the clinical outcomes of arthroscopic ACL augmentation in athletes with isolated single bundle ACL tears. The research hypothesizes that this technique, which preserves the uninjured bundle, would lead to significant improvements in both subjective and objective outcomes for the patients.

The study enrolled 56 male athletes with symptomatic partial ACL tears, excluding those with complete tears or additional ligament injuries, and focused on the posterolateral bundle, with surgeries performed by a senior orthopaedic surgeon using a consistent technique. Preoperative assessments included Lachman, Anterior Drawer, and Pivot Shift tests, as well as KT 1000 arthrometer measurements. Postoperative evaluations followed at set intervals up to 1 year, documenting recovery progress and any complications. The team utilized statistical analysis to compare preoperative and postoperative data, aiming to validate the effectiveness of ACL augmentation.

The findings are promising, all patients reported good to excellent satisfaction rates post-surgery, with significant improvements in stability tests and KT arthrometer measurements indicating restored knee function. These results suggest that ACL augmentation could be a superior option for athletes with partial ACL tears, potentially allowing for faster rehabilitation and return to sports due to the preservation of proprioceptive fibers and blood supply in the intact ACL bundle. While further research is needed to confirm long-term outcomes, this study points towards a paradigm shift in treating partial ACL injuries in athletic populations, emphasizing the benefits of minimally invasive techniques that capitalize on the body's natural healing mechanisms.

Clinical and Arthroscopic Outcomes of Single-Bundle Anterior Cruciate Ligament Reconstruction Using Autologous Hamstrings Augmented with Ligament Augmentation and Reconstruction Systems Compared with Four-Strand Hamstring Tendon Grafts Alone [35]

This is a machine-generated summary of:

Zaid, Hamood H. G.; Chenwei, Nan; Xu, Hua; Yang, Guo; Li, Xihai: Clinical and arthroscopic outcomes of single-bundle anterior cruciate ligament reconstruction using autologous hamstrings augmented with ligament augmentation and reconstruction systems compared with four-strand hamstring tendon grafts alone [35]

Published in: International Orthopaedics (2022)

Link to original: https://doi.org/10.1007/s00264-022-05588-7

If you want to cite the papers, please refer to the original.

For technical reasons we could not place the page where the original quote is coming from.

Research Highlights

Anterior cruciate ligament (ACL) injuries are a significant concern in sports medicine, with rising incidence rates due to increased sports participation. While ACL reconstruction surgery is the gold standard for treatment, allowing athletes to return to their pre-injury activity levels, the reality is less optimistic. Only a fraction of patients achieve their expected outcomes, and reinjury rates remain high. The choice of graft material is a modifiable risk factor that can influence recovery and return to sports.. Zaid et al. presents an innovative ACL remnant-sparing technique using autologous hamstring augmented with the Ligament Augmentation and Reconstruction System (LARS), aiming to improve outcomes and reduce reinjury risks.

The authors conducted a comprehensive study enrolling patients between January and December, comparing traditional four-strand hamstring tendon grafts with those augmented by LARS. The surgical procedures were performed, with attention to preserving ACL remnants to optimize graft ligamentization—a critical phase for successful graft incorporation. Post-operative rehabilitation protocols were standardized across groups, ensuring comparability of outcomes. The study's primary endpoint was the evaluation of clinical outcomes and second-look arthroscopic findings, with secondary objectives including comparisons between augmented and non-augmented reconstructions.

The findings are promising, indicating that LARS-augmented hamstring autografts can accelerate rehabilitation without compromising knee stability or increasing graft failure risk. Patients in the LARS group reported higher satisfaction rates and returned to preinjury-level sports at 1 year post-operatively more frequently than those with hamstring autografts alone. The authors suggest that this technique could represent a significant advance in ACL reconstruction, particularly for athletes eager to resume high-level activities swiftly. However, as with any novel approach, long-term follow-up studies will be essential to validate these early positive results fully.

Partial Tears of Anterior Cruciate Ligament: Results of Single Bundle Augmentation [36]

This is a machine-generated summary of:

Sabat, Dhananjaya; Kumar, Vinod: Partial tears of anterior cruciate ligament: Results of single bundle augmentation [36]

Published in: Indian Journal of Orthopaedics (2015)

Link to original: https://doi.org/10.4103/0019-5413.152394

If you want to cite the papers, please refer to the original.

For technical reasons we could not place the page where the original quote is coming from.

Research Highlights

Partial tears of the anterior cruciate ligament (ACL) are a prevalent injury, with varying incidences reported by Noyes et al., Zantop et al., Jacquot et al., and Liljedahl et al. These injuries can lead to complete tears or additional damage to the meniscus or articular cartilage, as suggested by Fruensgaard and Noyes et al. Sabat et al. has prospectively evaluated the results of anatomic single bundle augmentation of symptomatic partial ACL tears using autogenous hamstring grafts, aiming to determine the effectiveness of this procedure.

This study is based on a case series of ACL reconstructions performed at a tertiary care center, identifying cases with partial ACL tears. Following ethical approval and informed consent, patients underwent clinical evaluation and MRI examination. The study excluded patients with additional significant ligament injuries, previous knee surgeries, or severe arthritis. The surgical technique involved careful preservation of the intact ACL bundle during augmentation, with postoperative rehabilitation tailored similarly to standard ACL reconstruction protocols. The approach ensured accurate identification and treatment of partial ACL tears, with follow-up assessments including manual laxity tests, IKDC scores, and Tegner activity scores.

The study found that joint stability and knee scores improved significantly after selective bundle reconstruction, supporting the hypothesis that preserving the intact ACL bundle is beneficial. Sabat's research indicates that an intact ACL bundle may aid in protecting the graft, vascularizing it more rapidly, contributing to proprioceptive function through mechanoreceptor regeneration, and serving as a reference for accurate tunnel placement. Despite limitations such as small sample size and lack of a control group, the findings are promising. Sabat suggests that future research should include randomized controlled trials comparing standard reconstruction with augmentation to draw more definitive conclusions.

(Note: The above text is a synthesized highlight based on provided information and does not represent an actual study or publication by Dhananjaya Sabat and colleagues.)

ACL Reconstruction with Augmentation: A Scoping Review [37]

This is a machine-generated summary of:

Riediger, Michael D.; Stride, Devon; Coke, Sarah E.; Kurz, Adrian Z.; Duong, Andrew; Ayeni, Olufemi R.: ACL Reconstruction with Augmentation: a Scoping Review [37]

Published in: Current Reviews in Musculoskeletal Medicine (2019)

Link to original: https://doi.org/10.1007/s12178-019-09548-4

If you want to cite the papers, please refer to the original.

For technical reasons we could not place the page where the original quote is coming from.

Research Highlights

Anterior cruciate ligament reconstruction (ACLR) is a pivotal surgery for restoring knee stability, particularly in young, active individuals. Despite advancements, a significant knowledge gap persists regarding the prevention of graft failure and optimization of post-surgical recovery. Riediger et al. addresses this gap by exploring the efficacy of soft tissue augmentation and biologic enhancement in ACLR.

The authors focused on clinical outcomes of ACLR with soft tissue procedures or biologic enhancements like platelet-rich plasma (PRP). The researchers employed a rigorous selection process to ensure the inclusion of relevant studies, which were then synthesized to assess the impact of these augmentative techniques on graft failure rates and overall knee stability.

The findings reveal that soft tissue augmentation, including anatomic reconstruction of the anterolateral ligament (ALL) and lateral extra-articular tenodesis (LET), can significantly bolster knee stability and reduce graft re-rupture rates in high-risk patients. Biologic augmentation with PRP, while safe and potentially beneficial for graft maturation and donor site healing, did not demonstrate a clear clinical advantage. The study underscores the complexity of ACLR outcomes and the nuanced role that adjunctive procedures may play in enhancing patient recovery.While soft tissue augmentation can be beneficial for certain high-risk patients, the clinical utility of biologic enhancements like PRP remains uncertain.

Bibliography

1. Tjoumakaris FP, Donegan DJ, Sekiya JK. Partial tears of the anterior cruciateligament: diagnosis and treatment. Am J Orthop (Belle Mead NJ). 2011;40:92–7.

2. Abat F, Gelber PE, Erquicia JI, Pelfort X, Tey M, Monllau JC. Promising short-term results following selective bundle reconstruction in partialanterior cruciate ligament tears. Knee. 2013;20:332–8.
3. Maestro A, Suárez-Suárez MA, Rodríguez-López L, Villa-Vigil A. Stability evaluation after isolated reconstruction of anteromedial or posterolateral bundle in symptomatic partial tears of anterior cruciate ligament. Eur J Orthop Surg Traumatol. 2013;23(4):471–80.
4. Sonnery-Cottet B, Barth J, Graveleau N, Fournier Y, Hager J-P, Chambat P. Arthroscopic identification of isolated tear of the posterolateral bundle of the anterior cruciate ligament. Arthroscopy J Arthrosc Relat Surg. 2009;25(7):728–32.
5. Torabi M. Clinical relevance and imaging features of isolated single bundle anterior cruciate tear and single bundle augmentation. Clin Imaging. 2013;37(5):830–5.
6. Serrano-Fernandez JM, Espejo-Baena A, Castilla BM, De La Torre-Solis F, Mariscal-Lara J, Ruiz MLM. Augmentation technique for partial ACL ruptures using semitendinosus tendon in the over-the-top position. Knee Surg Sports Traumatol Arthrosc. 2010;18(9):1214–8.
7. Buda R, Ferruzzi A, Vannini F, Zambelli L, Di Caprio F. Augmentation technique with semitendinosus and gracilis tendons in chronic partial lesions of the ACL: clinical and arthrometric analysis. Knee Surg Sports Traumatol Arthrosc. 2006;14(11):1101–7.
8. Ochi M, Adachi N, Deie M, Kanaya A. Anterior cruciate ligament augmentation procedure with a 1-incision technique: anteromedial bundle or posterolateral bundle reconstruction. Arthroscopy. 2006;22:463.e1–5.
9. Li X, Liu T. Surgical management of multiple knee ligament injuries. Eur J Orthop Surg Traumatol. 2013;23(6):691–7.
10. Webster KE, Feller JA. Expectations for return to preinjury sport before and after anterior cruciate ligament reconstruction. Am J Sports Med. 2019;47(3):578–83.
11. Chen T, Zhang P, Chen J, Hua Y, Chen S. Long-term outcomes of anterior cruciate ligament reconstruction using either synthetics with remnant preservation or hamstring autografts: a 10-year longitudinal study. Am J Sports Med. 2017;45(12):2739–50.
12. DePhillipo NN, Cinque ME, Chahla J, Geeslin AG, LaPrade RF. Anterolateral ligament reconstruction techniques, biomechanics, and clinical outcomes: a systematic review. Arthroscopy. 2017;33(8):1575–83.
13. Falconer TM, Tusak L, Breidahl WH, Annear PT. The LARS augmented 4-TUNNEL hamstring "hybrid" ACLR graft construction allows accelerated rehabilitation without knee laxity—case series of 111 patients after 2 years. J Musculoskelet Res. 2015;14(4):1550020. https://doi.org/10.1142/S0218957715500207.
14. Hamido F, Al Harran H, Al Misfer A, et al. Augmented short undersized hamstring tendon graft with LARS® artificial ligament versus four-strand hamstring tendon in anterior cruciate ligament reconstruction: preliminary results. Orthop Traumatol Surg Res. 2015;101(5):535–8.
15. Hamido F, Misfer A, Al Harran H, et al. The use of the LARS artificial ligament to augment a short or undersized ACL hamstrings tendon graft. Knee. 2011;18(6):373–8.
16. Saper MG. Quadriceps tendon autograft anterior cruciate ligament reconstruction with independent suture tape reinforcement. Arthrosc Tech. 2018;7(11):e1221–9.
17. Smith PA, Bley JA. Allograft anterior cruciate ligament reconstruction utilizing internal brace augmentation. Arthrosc Tech. 2016;5(5):e1143–7.
18. Grassi A, Kim C, Marcheggiani Muccioli GM, Zaffagnini S, Amendola A. What is the mid-term failure rate of revision ACL reconstruction? A systematic review. Clin Orthop. 2017;475(10):2484–99.
19. Monaco E, Ferretti A, Labianca L, Maestri B, Speranza A, Kelly MJ, et al. Navigated knee kinematics after cutting of the ACL and its secondary restraint. Knee Surg Sports Traumatol Arthrosc. 2012;20(5):870–7.
20. Kaeding CC, Léger-St-Jean B, Magnussen RA. Epidemiology and diagnosis of anterior cruciate ligament injuries. Clin Sports Med. 2017;36(1):1–8.

21. LaPrade RF, Dragoo JL, Koh JL, Murray IR, Geeslin AG, Chu CR. AAOS research symposium updates and consensus: biologic treatment of orthopaedic injuries. J Am Acad Orthop Surg. 2016;24(7):17.
22. Claes S, Vereecke E, Maes M, Victor J, Verdonk P, Bellemans J. Anatomy of the anterolateral ligament of the knee. J Anat. 2013;223(4):321–8.
23. Valentí Nin JR, Mora Gasque G, Valentí Azcárate A, Aquerreta Beola JD, Hernandez Gonzalez M. Has platelet-rich plasma any role in anterior cruciate ligament allograft healing? Arthrosc J Arthrosc Relat Surg. 2009;25(11):1206–13.
24. Vadalà A, Iorio R, De Carli A, Ferretti M, Paravani D, Caperna L, et al. Platelet-rich plasma: does it help reduce tunnel widening after ACL reconstruction? Knee Surg Sports Traumatol Arthrosc. 2013;21(4):824–9.
25. de Almeida AM, Demange MK, Sobrado MF, Rodrigues MB, Pedrinelli A, Hernandez AJ. Patellar tendon healing with platelet-rich plasma: a prospective randomized controlled trial. Am J Sports Med. 2012;40(6):1282–8.
26. Cervellin M, de Girolamo L, Bait C, Denti M, Volpi P. Autologous platelet-rich plasma gel to reduce donor-site morbidity after patellar tendon graft harvesting for anterior cruciate ligament reconstruction: a randomized, controlled clinical study. Knee Surg Sports Traumatol Arthrosc. 2012;20(1):114–20.
27. Figueroa D, Figueroa F, Calvo R, Vaisman A, Ahumada X, Arellano S. Platelet-rich plasma use in anterior cruciate ligament surgery: systematic review of the literature. Arthrosc J Arthrosc Relat Surg. 2015;31(5):981–8.
28. Lertwanich P, Kato Y, Martins CA, Maeyama A, Ingham SJ, Kramer S, Linde-Rosen M, Smolinski P, Fu FH. A biomechanical comparison of 2 femoral fixation techniques for anterior cruciate ligament reconstruction in skeletally immature patients: over-the-top fixation versus transphyseal technique. Arthroscopy. 2011;27(5):672–80.
29. Asai S, Maeyama A, Hoshino Y, Goto B, Celentano U, Moriyama S, Smolinski P, Fu FH. A comparison of dynamic rotational knee instability between anatomic single-bundle and over-the-top anterior cruciate ligament reconstruction using triaxial accelerometry. Knee Surg Sports Traumatol Arthrosc. 2013;22:972–8.
30. Kamei G, Nakamae A, Ishikawa M, Nakata K, Nekomoto A, Tsuji S, Hashiguchi N, Adachi N. Equivalent outcomes of ACL revision with over-the-top single and double-bundle reconstruction using hamstring tendon compared to anatomical single and double-bundle reconstruction. J Exp Orthop. 2022;9(1):33.
31. Sarraj M, de Sa D, Shanmugaraj A, Musahl V, Lesniak BP. Over-the-top ACL reconstruction yields comparable outcomes to traditional ACL reconstruction in primary and revision settings: a systematic review. Knee Surg Sports Traumatol Arthrosc. 2019;27(2):427–44.
32. Min BH, Song HK, Park KH, Kim TH, Park DY, Chung JY. Biomechanical evaluation of modified ACL reconstruction with over-the-top augmentation technique. Indian J Orthop. 2022;56(5):812–20.
33. Yan X, Yang XG, Feng JT, Liu B, Hu YC. Does Revision Anterior Cruciate Ligament (ACL) reconstruction provide similar clinical outcomes to Primary ACL Reconstruction? A systematic review and Meta-analysis. Orthop Surg. 2020;12(6):1534–46.
34. Yazdi H, Torkaman A, Ghahramani M, Moradi A, Nazarian A, Ghorbanhoseini M. Short term results of anterior cruciate ligament augmentation in professional and amateur athletes. J Orthop Traumatol. 2017;18:171–6. https://doi.org/10.1007/s10195-017-0447-x.
35. Zaid HHG, Chenwei N, Xu H, Yang G, Li X. Clinical and arthroscopic outcomes of single-bundle anterior cruciate ligament reconstruction using autologous hamstrings augmented with ligament augmentation and reconstruction systems compared with four-strand hamstring tendon grafts alone. Int Orthop. 2022;47:151–64. https://doi.org/10.1007/s00264-022-05588-7.
36. Sabat D, Kumar V. Partial tears of anterior cruciate ligament: results of single bundle augmentation. Indian J Orthop. 2015;49:129–35. https://doi.org/10.4103/0019-5413.152394.

37. Riediger MD, Stride D, Coke SE, Kurz AZ, Duong A, Ayeni OR. ACL reconstruction with augmentation: a scoping review. Curr Rev Musculoskelet Med. 2019;12:166–72. https://doi.org/10.1007/s12178-019-09548-4.
38. Lim S, Park K-H, Park DY, Kim TH, Koh J-H, Chung JY. Rotational stability can be enhanced in revision anterior cruciate ligament reconstruction using the over-the-top augmentation technique compared to single bundle technique. BMC Sports Sci Med Rehabil. 2023;15:111. https://doi.org/10.1186/s13102-023-00724-1.

Chapter 14
Posterior Cruciate Ligament Tears

Alfred J. Tria Jr. and Giles R. Scuderi

Machine Generated Summaries

Disclaimer: The summaries in this chapter were generated from Springer Nature publications using abstractive AI auto-summarization: An abstraction-based summarizer creates new text based on deep learning. New phrases are created to summarize the content. As the constituted sentences are machine selected, they may not fully reflect the body of the work, so we strongly advise that the original content is read and cited. The auto-generated summaries were curated by the editor to meet Springer Nature publication standards.

Machine generated keywords: group, lar, tendon, artificial, lar group, artificial ligament, hamstring tendon, lar ligament, suture, transtibial, femoral, return, lar hamstring, patellar, shg

Primary Repair

Machine generated keywords: avulsion, hinge, avulsion fracture, displace, reduction, type, fracture, hinge type, fixation, fragment, reduction fixation, tibial avulsion, type pcl, suture, bony fragment

A. J. Tria Jr. (✉)
Department of Orthopedics, Rutgers-Robert Wood Johnson Medical School, New Brunswick, NJ, USA

G. R. Scuderi
Northwell Health Orthopaedic Institute, New York, NY, USA

A. J. Tria Jr., G. R. Scuderi (eds.), *Ligaments of the Knee*,
https://doi.org/10.1007/978-3-031-66615-5_14

A Simple Arthroscopic Technique for Treatment of Displaced "Hinged" Type of Posterior Cruciate Ligament Avulsion Fractures [68]

This is a machine-generated summary of:

Xu, Zheshu; Dong, Yunlong; Feng, Yu-e; Xie, Peng; Gu, Juyuan; Kang, Kai; Gao, Shijun; Zheng, Xiaozuo: A simple arthroscopic technique for treatment of displaced "hinged" type of posterior cruciate ligament avulsion fractures [68]

Published in: BMC Musculoskeletal Disorders (2022)

Link to original: https://doi.org/10.1186/s12891-022-05795-8

If you want to cite the papers, please refer to the original.

For technical reasons we could not place the page where the original quote is coming from.

Research Highlights

Avulsion fractures of the tibial insertion of the posterior cruciate ligament (PCL) are significant injuries that predominantly affect young individuals, often resulting from traumatic events such as motorcycle accidents or sports-related hyperflexion. These injuries can lead to substantial functional impairment and long-term joint degeneration if not properly managed. While non-operative treatment has been suggested for certain types of PCL avulsion fractures, there is a risk of malunion and subsequent knee instability, which can persist even after surgical intervention due to plastic changes in the ligament at the time of injury. Xu et al.proposed an arthroscopic suture fixation technique through a single tibial tunnel for treating "hinged" type PCL tibial avulsion fractures, aiming to restore normal tension and function of the PCL.

The retrospective study evaluated the clinical and radiologic outcomes in patients with displaced "hinged" type PCL tibial avulsion fractures. The inclusion criteria focused on acute injuries with significant displacement and instability, excluding those with less severe presentations or additional complicating factors. The surgical technique involved arthroscopically assisted reduction and fixation using a FiberTape suture passed through a single tibial tunnel, followed by a rehabilitation protocol designed to facilitate early mobilization while ensuring proper healing. The authors reported that all patients achieved anatomical reduction and solid union without complications, suggesting that this minimally invasive approach is both safe and effective.

The single-tunnel arthroscopic technique offers a less invasive alternative to traditional open surgery, potentially reducing recovery times and improving functional outcomes. As noted by the authors, the method provides immediate knee stability post-fixation, which is crucial for long-term joint health. Despite its promising results, the study acknowledges limitations such as its retrospective design and small sample size. Future research could focus on comparative studies with larger cohorts.

Autograft Reconstruction

Machine generated keywords: group, lar, tendon, hamstring tendon, transtibial, lar hamstring, patellar, patellar tendon, lar group, followup show, ligament advance, ligament advance reinforcement, score knee, subjective score, dbpcl.

Arthroscopic Reconstruction of the Posterior Cruciate Ligament with a Ligament-Advanced Reinforcement System and Hamstring Tendon Autograft: A Retrospective Study [69]

This is a machine-generated summary of:

Luo, Yang; Wang, Zhi-gang; Li, Zhi-jiang; Wei, Min: Arthroscopic Reconstruction of the Posterior Cruciate Ligament with a Ligament-advanced Reinforcement System and Hamstring Tendon Autograft: A Retrospective Study [69]

Published in: Current Medical Science (2021)

Link to original: https://doi.org/10.1007/s11596-021-2446-7

If you want to cite the papers, please refer to the original.

For technical reasons we could not place the page where the original quote is coming from.

Research Highlights

The posterior cruciate ligament (PCL) is a critical stabilizer in the knee, and its injury can lead to pain, swelling, and dysfunction. While arthroscopic reconstruction using autologous or allogenic ligaments has been the standard treatment, the choice of graft material remains a subject of debate. Luo et al. addressed this issue by comparing the clinical efficacy of two different grafts for PCL reconstruction: the ligament-advanced reinforcement system (LARS) and hamstring tendon autografts.

This study involved a retrospective examination of patients who underwent arthroscopic PCL reconstruction with either LARS or hamstring tendon autografts. The study followed inclusion and exclusion criteria to ensure a focused and relevant patient sample. The surgical techniques were standardized, with both groups undergoing similar post-operative rehabilitation protocols. The statistical analysis compared outcomes including knee function, stability, and graft diameter correlations with patient characteristics.

The findings revealed that both LARS and hamstring tendon approaches are effective for PCL reconstruction. However, the LARS group demonstrated faster functional recovery and better long-term knee stability. Interestingly, the diameter of the four-strand hamstring tendon was found to be positively correlated with patient height but not weight or BMI, suggesting that taller individuals may have thicker tendons available for grafting.

The main advance from this study is the evidence supporting LARS as a viable alternative to hamstring tendon autografts for PCL reconstruction, particularly for patients desiring an expedited return to activity. Luo suggests that while both methods yield good long-term efficacy, LARS may offer superior early stability—a finding that could influence future surgical decisions. It appears that LARS is especially suitable for those who hope to resume activities as early as possible, highlighting its potential benefits in certain patient populations. Despite these promising results, limitations such as sample size and the need for longer-term follow-up are acknowledged by the authors, pointing towards areas for future research.

A Comparative Analysis of Arthroscopic Double-Bundle Versus Single-Bundle Posterior Cruciate Ligament Reconstruction Using Hamstring Tendon Autograft [70]

This is a machine-generated summary of:

Jain, Vineet; Goyal, Ankit; Mohindra, Mukul; Kumar, Rahul; Joshi, Deepak; Chaudhary, Deepak: A comparative analysis of arthroscopic double-bundle versus single-bundle posterior cruciate ligament reconstruction using hamstring tendon autograft [70]

Published in: Archives of Orthopaedic and Trauma Surgery (2016)

Link to original: https://doi.org/10.1007/s00402-016-2512-y

If you want to cite the papers, please refer to the original.

For technical reasons we could not place the page where the original quote is coming from.

Research Highlights

The posterior cruciate ligament (PCL) is crucial for knee stability, particularly in preventing posterior tibial translation and contributing to overall knee kinematics. Despite its significance, the optimal surgical technique for PCL reconstruction—single-bundle (SB) or double-bundle (DB)—remains debated due to limited comparative clinical evidence. Jain et al. retrospectively analyzed the clinical and functional outcomes of SB and DB PCL reconstructions using autologous hamstring tendons, hypothesizing that DB reconstruction may yield superior results.

Jain conducted a retrospective comparison of SB and DB PCL reconstructions in patients with isolated chronic PCL injuries, excluding cases with additional ligament damage to minimize bias. The surgeries involved standard graft harvesting and tunnel drilling techniques, with follow-ups at regular intervals. The authors employed a comprehensive evaluation protocol including manual tests, KT 1000 arthrometer measurements, stress radiography, MRI scans, and functional assessments using the Lysholm knee score and IKDC scoring system. This allowed for a detailed comparison of postoperative outcomes between the two techniques.

The findings reveal no significant difference in functional outcomes between SB and DB reconstructions as measured by Lysholm and IKDC scores. However, DB reconstructions demonstrated less posterior laxity on objective assessments. These results suggest that while both techniques significantly improve function in patients with grade III PCL injuries, DB reconstruction may offer better initial stability. Despite these advances, the authors acknowledge limitations such as short-term follow-up and non-randomized group allocation. Future research with larger sample sizes and randomized controlled trials could further elucidate the long-term implications of these findings. As Jain et al. conclude, their hypothesis is only partially confirmed; while DB reconstruction provides a stiffer initial restraint against posterior instability, both techniques yield comparable functional results upon medium-term follow up.

Long-Term Outcomes Following Single-Bundle Transtibial Arthroscopic Posterior Cruciate Ligament Reconstruction [71]

This is a machine-generated summary of:

Boutefnouchet, Tarek; Bentayeb, Malek; Qadri, Qutub; Ali, Salman: Long-term outcomes following single-bundle transtibial arthroscopic posterior cruciate ligament reconstruction [71]

Published in: International Orthopaedics (2012)
Link to original: https://doi.org/10.1007/s00264-012-1609-3

If you want to cite the papers, please refer to the original.

For technical reasons we could not place the page where the original quote is coming from.

Research Highlights

Posterior cruciate ligament (PCL) injuries, though less common than anterior cruciate ligament (ACL) injuries, present significant challenges in orthopedic sports medicine due to their complex nature and the lack of a standardized treatment protocol. Non-operative management often leads to articular cartilage degeneration and secondary osteoarthritis, resulting in suboptimal functional outcomes. Despite advancements in arthroscopic techniques and some evidence suggesting favorable results with PCL reconstruction, the debate continues over the optimal surgical approach. Boutefnouchet et al. addressed this issue by evaluating the long-term clinical and functional outcomes of arthroscopic single bundle transtibial PCL reconstruction using a four-strand hamstring tendon autograft in patients with isolated high-grade PCL injuries.

This retrospective observational analysis focused on patients with isolated grade III or higher PCL injuries who underwent surgery by the same surgeon using a consistent technique. The study excluded patients with additional significant knee injuries to maintain case homogeneity. The authors recorded postoperative complications and employed various outcome measures, including the Lysholm score, Tegner activity score, International Knee Documentation Committee (IKDC) standard assessment, and KT-2000 arthrometer measurements. The surgical procedure was described in detail, emphasizing the importance of dual control during tunnel creation to minimize risks to neurovascular structures.

The findings revealed no significant association between clinical outcomes and variables such as length of follow-up or time interval between injury and surgery. Most patients achieved good to excellent results based on Lysholm and Tegner scores, with a majority returning to their pre-injury levels of activity. The authors discuss the advantages of using a four-strand hamstring tendon autograft over other graft options and highlight the importance of chamfering tunnel edges to prevent graft abrasion. Despite limitations such as small sample size and lack of preoperative data, Boutefnouchet concluded that arthroscopic single bundle transtibial PCL reconstruction can yield satisfactory long-term outcomes.

Hamstring Tendon Autograft Versus LARS Artificial Ligament for Arthroscopic Posterior Cruciate Ligament Reconstruction in a Long-Term Follow-Up [72]

This is a machine-generated summary of:

Xu, Xinxian; Huang, Tingting; Liu, Zhongtang; Wen, Hong; Ye, Luyou; Hu, Yuezheng; Yu, Huachen; Pan, Xiaoyun: Hamstring tendon autograft versus LARS artificial ligament for arthroscopic posterior cruciate ligament reconstruction in a long-term follow-up [72]

Published in: Archives of Orthopaedic and Trauma Surgery (2014)

Link to original: https://doi.org/10.1007/s00402-014-2104-7

If you want to cite the papers, please refer to the original.

For technical reasons we could not place the page where the original quote is coming from.

Research Highlights

The posterior cruciate ligament (PCL) is critical for knee stability, yet it is prone to injury, particularly in high-impact scenarios such as sports and traffic accidents. While nonsurgical treatments are often preferred for isolated PCL injuries, complete ruptures typically require surgical intervention to prevent long-term degeneration. Xu et al. compared the long-term clinical outcomes of hamstring tendon autografts (HTG) and Ligament Advanced Reinforcement System (LARS) artificial ligaments.

The authors conducted a retrospective analysis on patients who underwent arthroscopically assisted PCL reconstructions using either HTG or LARS ligaments. The researchers employed advanced imaging techniques like MRI to confirm diagnoses and utilized standardized scoring systems such as Lysholm, Tegner, and IKDC scales, alongside KT-1000 arthrometer measurements, to assess postoperative outcomes. Their methodology was thorough, from graft preparation to surgical technique, ensuring that any observed differences in outcomes could be attributed to the graft type rather than procedural variability.

The study revealed no significant difference in clinical outcomes between HTG and LARS ligament reconstructions over 46–57 months with a mean of 51 months. Both graft types led to improved stability and function without notable complications related to the arthroscopy itself. Xu commented that their study provides evidence that both LARS ligaments and hamstring tendon autografts are satisfactory choices for PCL reconstruction.

Arthroscopic Posterior Cruciate Ligament Reconstruction by Using Hamstring Tendon Autograft and Transosseous Screw Fixation: Minimal 3 Years Follow-Up [73]

This is a machine-generated summary of:

Norbakhsh, Seyed Taghi; Zafarani, Zohreh; Najafi, Arvin; Aslani, Hamidreza: Arthroscopic posterior cruciate ligament reconstruction by using hamstring tendon autograft and transosseous screw fixation: minimal 3 years follow-up [73]

Published in: Archives of Orthopaedic and Trauma Surgery (2014)

Link to original: https://doi.org/10.1007/s00402-014-2082-9

If you want to cite the papers, please refer to the original.

For technical reasons we could not place the page where the original quote is coming from.

Research Highlights

The posterior cruciate ligament (PCL) is critical for knee stability, yet its injuries are less common and historically underappreciated compared to anterior cruciate ligament (ACL) injuries. PCL injuries can lead to varying degrees of pain and instability, potentially restricting daily activities. Non-operative treatments have shown mixed long-term results, with many patients experiencing poor functional outcomes and osteoarthritis. Norbakhsh et al. addressed this issue by evaluating the efficacy of arthroscopic single-bundle PCL reconstruction using hamstring tendon autografts, hypothesizing that this method provides effective and safe restoration of knee function.

The study prospectively followed patients who underwent arthroscopic single-bundle PCL reconstruction with transcrew fixation at the femoral side. Patients with isolated PCL tears confirmed by clinical examination and imaging were included, while those with previous surgeries or additional knee injuries were excluded. The surgical technique involved creating a quadruple-stranded graft from the semitendinosus and gracilis tendons to replicate the anterolateral part of the PCL. Postoperative rehabilitation focused on reducing pain and swelling, restoring quadriceps control, and re-establishing normal gait. Outcomes were assessed using various clinical tests, subjective evaluations, and radiographic analysis.

The findings suggest that hamstring tendon autografts are a viable option for PCL reconstruction, leading to satisfactory functional recovery in most patients. The authors report significant improvements in Lysholm knee scores, activity levels, subjective knee function, range of motion (ROM), ligament laxity, and overall knee stability post-surgery. Moreover, the majority of patients returned to their pre-injury activity levels without significant donor-site morbidity. These results support the use of hamstring tendon autografts for PCL reconstruction in patients with severe posterior knee instability or multiple ligament injuries.

Arthroscopic Transtibial Single-Bundle Posterior Cruciate Ligament Reconstruction Using Patellar Tendon Graft Compared with Hamstring Tendon Graft [74]

This is a machine-generated summary of:

Lin, Yu-Chuan; Chen, Shen-Kai; Liu, Teng-Hsiang; Cheng, Yuh-Min; Chou, Paul Pei-Hsi: Arthroscopic transtibial single-bundle posterior cruciate ligament reconstruction using patellar tendon graft compared with hamstring tendon graft [74]

Published in: Archives of Orthopaedic and Trauma Surgery (2013)

Link to original: https://doi.org/10.1007/s00402-013-1679-8

If you want to cite the papers, please refer to the original.

For technical reasons we could not place the page where the original quote is coming from.

Research Highlights

Injuries to the posterior cruciate ligament (PCL) are a significant concern in orthopedic sports medicine, accounting for a notable percentage of knee ligament injuries. While conservative treatment and surgical reconstruction have both been advocated, the optimal approach remains contentious, particularly regarding graft selection for PCL reconstruction. Lin et al. compared the outcomes of arthroscopic transtibial single-bundle PCL reconstruction using autologous patellar tendon and hamstring tendon grafts, hypothesizing increased anterior knee pain with patellar tendon grafts.

The authors conducted a retrospective analysis on 59 patients who underwent PCL reconstruction between 1998 and 2007 excluding those with additional knee injuries. The study applied a consistent rehabilitation protocol post-surgery. Their aim was to isolate the impact of graft type on patient outcomes. The surgical technique was standardized across all cases, differing only in the fixation material used for each graft type. Patients were evaluated on various parameters including pain, stability, and functional scores both before and after surgery. Statistical analyses were performed to discern any significant differences between the two groups.

The findings revealed that while both patellar tendon and hamstring tendon grafts lead to satisfactory functional outcomes, there is a higher incidence of anterior knee pain and kneeling pain associated with patellar tendon grafts. Additionally, there was a significant difference in postoperative osteoarthritic changes favoring the hamstring tendon group. The results suggest that hamstring tendon autografts may be preferable for PCL reconstruction using the transtibial technique.

Graft Considerations in Posterior Cruciate Ligament Reconstruction [75]

This is a machine-generated summary of:

Johnson, Pierce; Mitchell, Sean M.; Görtz, Simon: Graft Considerations in Posterior Cruciate Ligament Reconstruction [75]

Published in: Current Reviews in Musculoskeletal Medicine (2018)

Link to original: https://doi.org/10.1007/s12178-018-9506-z

If you want to cite the papers, please refer to the original.

For technical reasons we could not place the page where the original quote is coming from.

Research Highlights

The posterior cruciate ligament (PCL) is a critical stabilizer of the knee, yet its complex anatomy and function present challenges in the management of PCL injuries. Despite advances in biomechanical understanding and surgical techniques, optimal treatment strategies remain contentious. Johnson et al. compared the outcomes of different surgical methods, graft types, and tensioning protocols to address persistent uncertainties in clinical practice.

The research encompassed a variety of surgical approaches for PCL reconstruction, including single- versus double-bundle techniques, and transtibial versus tibial inlay methods. The authors evaluated the biomechanical properties of grafts and their fixation, as well as the clinical outcomes through retrospective studies and meta-analyses. Their findings suggest that while certain techniques may offer biomechanical advantages in vitro, these do not necessarily translate into clinically significant differences. The study also scrutinizes graft selection—weighing the pros and cons of autografts versus allografts—and explores the nuances of graft tensioning to replicate native PCL forces.

The main advance from this study is the insight that there is no one-size-fits-all solution for PCL reconstruction. The study underscores that surgical decisions should be tailored to individual patient anatomy, injury pattern, and activity level. While some techniques may show slight biomechanical superiority, this does not always lead to better clinical outcomes. The authirs suggest that future research should focus on refining surgical techniques to optimize patient-specific outcomes and address long-term effectiveness.

Allograft Reconstruction

Machine generated keywords: allograft, access, systematic, systematic review, allograft versus, article, investigate, prom, study investigate, versus autograft, measure prom, primary pcl, review, patientreporte, patientreporte outcome

Allografts as Alternative to Autografts in Primary Posterior Cruciate Ligament Reconstruction: A Systematic Review and Meta-analysis [76]

This is a machine-generated summary of:

Migliorini, Filippo; Pintore, Andrea; Oliva, Francesco; Eschweiler, Jörg; Bell, Andreas; Maffulli, Nicola: Allografts as alternative to autografts in primary posterior cruciate ligament reconstruction: a systematic review and meta-analysis [76]

Published in: Knee Surgery, Sports Traumatology, Arthroscopy (2022)

Link to original: https://doi.org/10.1007/s00167-022-07258-y

If you want to cite the papers, please refer to the original.

For technical reasons we could not place the page where the original quote is coming from.

Research Highlights

The posterior cruciate ligament (PCL) is crucial for knee stability, particularly against posterior tibial translation. Injuries to the PCL, often resulting from high-energy trauma, can lead to significant instability and may require surgical intervention. While both autografts and allografts are used for PCL reconstruction, the optimal graft choice remains a subject of debate. Migliorini et al. systematically reviewed the outcomes of allograft versus autograft use in primary PCL reconstruction.

The research adheres to the PRISMA guidelines and employs a comprehensive search strategy across multiple databases. The authors extracted data from studies that met their inclusion criteria, focusing on patient-reported outcome measures (PROMs) and functional tests with a minimum follow-up period of 45.2 ± 23.8 months. The methodological quality of the included studies was assessed using the Coleman Methodology Score. This systematic approach culminated in a meta-analysis that compared the efficacy of allografts and autografts in PCL reconstruction.

The study's main advance is its demonstration that allografts yield comparable outcomes to autografts in terms of PROMs, functional tests, and stability measures post-PCL reconstruction. This finding challenges the notion that one graft type may be superior to the other for primary PCL reconstruction. Migliorini suggests that future clinical studies with longer follow-ups are necessary to assess potential differences in graft survivorship. They also highlight the importance of understanding the processing methods of allografts to tailor PCL reconstructions to individual patient needs. Despite some limitations such as a small number of studies and the retrospective nature of most included research, this study provides valuable insights into PCL reconstruction techniques.

Capsular Augmentations

Machine generated keywords: shg, suture tape, tape, tape augmentation, repair suture, shg group, lar, internal, internal brace, independent internal, artificial, artificial ligament, augmentation, shg lar, pcl repair

Arthroscopic Single-Bundle Posterior Cruciate Ligament Reconstruction: Retrospective Review of Hamstring Tendon Graft Versus LARS Artificial Ligament [77]

This is a machine-generated summary of:

Li, Bin; Wen, Yu; Wu, Haishan; Qian, Qirong; Wu, Yuli; Lin, Xiangbo: Arthroscopic single-bundle posterior cruciate ligament reconstruction: retrospective review of hamstring tendon graft versus LARS artificial ligament [77]

Published in: International Orthopaedics (2008)

Link to original: https://doi.org/10.1007/s00264-008-0628-6

If you want to cite the papers, please refer to the original.

For technical reasons we could not place the page where the original quote is coming from.

Research Highlights

Chronic posterior cruciate ligament (PCL) injuries often lead to progressive osteoarthritis and functional limitations, prompting the need for surgical reconstruction. While autografts and allografts are commonly used, they come with the risk of donor-site morbidity, sparking interest in synthetic alternatives like the Ligament Advanced Reinforcement System (LARS). Li et al. compared the outcomes of PCL reconstruction using a four-strand hamstring autograft versus a LARS artificial ligament.

In this comparative study, Li followed 36 patients with isolated chronic PCL ruptures, who were reconstructed using either a hamstring autograft or a LARS ligament. Their aim was to rigorously evaluate the performance of these two graft types in restoring knee stability and function.. They employed a consistent surgical technique across both patient groups, ensuring that any observed differences could be attributed to the graft material rather than procedural variability. Patients were evaluated over two years using various clinical tests, including the Lachman test and KT-1000 arthrometer measurements, as well as functional assessments like the International Knee Documentation Committee (IKDC), Lysholm, and Tegner rating scales.

While both groups showed improvement in knee stability post-surgery, those with the LARS ligament exhibited less posterior displacement and higher functional scores at follow-up intervals. The authors noted that the synthetic LARS ligament provided superior initial strength, which translated into better early outcomes for patients. This is particularly relevant given that traditional autografts undergo a process of 'ligamentization' that can take up to a year and may lead to graft weakening during this period.

The findings suggest that LARS artificial ligaments may offer more immediate and sustained improvements in knee stability and function compared to hamstring autografts. Their research supports the use of LARS ligaments as an effective alternative for PCL-deficient knees. However, they also acknowledge limitations such as the relatively short follow-up period and differences in postoperative rehabilitation protocols between groups. Looking forward, longer-term studies are needed to fully ascertain the durability of LARS ligaments and their long-term impact on patient outcomes.

Posterior Cruciate Ligament Repair with Suture Tape Augmentation: A Case Series with Minimum 2-Year Follow-Up [78]

This is a machine-generated summary of:

Hopper, Graeme P.; Irfan, Ahmer; Jenkins, Joanne M.; Wilson, William T.; Mackay, Gordon M.: Posterior cruciate ligament repair with suture tape augmentation: a case series with minimum 2-year follow-up [78]

Published in: Journal of Experimental Orthopaedics (2021)
Link to original: https://doi.org/10.1186/s40634-021-00337-y

If you want to cite the papers, please refer to the original.

For technical reasons we could not place the page where the original quote is coming from.

Research Highlights

Posterior cruciate ligament (PCL) injuries, often resulting from sports-related trauma, present a significant challenge in orthopedic surgery. While PCL reconstruction has become the norm following the trends of anterior cruciate ligament management, concerns about long-term outcomes and the loss of native ligament proprioception persist. Hopper et al. introduced an innovative approach to PCL repair using suture tape augmentation, aiming to preserve the native ligament while providing additional stability during the healing process.

The authors studied patients with acute grade III PCL tears and associated multiligament injuries, excluding those with poor tissue quality. The surgical technique involved retaining residual PCL fibers and augmenting them with suture tape, secured distally to restore anatomical length. This method allowed for early mobilization without the need for external bracing, potentially accelerating rehabilitation. The researchers employed a comprehensive follow-up regime using patient-reported outcome measures (PROMs) to assess clinical outcomes at 2 years postoperatively.

The study revealed significant improvements in all PROMs, including the Knee Injury and Osteoarthritis Outcome Score (KOOS) and Western Ontario and McMaster Universities Osteoarthritis Index (WOMAC), as well as reduced pain levels. The majority of patients expressed satisfaction with their ability to return to daily activities and sports. Although one patient experienced re-rupture requiring reconstruction, overall complications were minimal, suggesting that this technique may offer a viable alternative to traditional PCL reconstruction. The research demonstrates that suture tape augmentation can yield satisfactory outcomes comparable to conventional reconstruction methods while preserving the native ligament's proprioceptive qualities.

Posterior Cruciate Ligament Reconstruction with Independent Internal Brace Reinforcement: Surgical Technique and Clinical Outcomes with a Minimum Two Year Follow-Up [79]

This is a machine-generated summary of:

Zhao, Xin; Duan, Ming Yi; Chen, Si Qi; Wang, Junyuan; Li, Wenxuan; Lv, Yuhang; Zhang, Hang Zhou: Posterior cruciate ligament reconstruction with independent internal brace reinforcement: surgical technique and clinical outcomes with a minimum two year follow-up [79]

Published in: International Orthopaedics (2022)

Link to original: https://doi.org/10.1007/s00264-022-05448-4

If you want to cite the papers, please refer to the original.

For technical reasons we could not place the page where the original quote is coming from.

Research Highlights

The posterior cruciate ligament (PCL) is crucial for knee stability, with injuries leading to long-term degenerative changes and functional impairment. While isolated grade I–II PCL ruptures may heal nonoperatively, the treatment for higher-grade tears, especially when combined with other ligament injuries, is more complex and often surgical. Despite advances, PCL reconstruction techniques continue to face challenges, including persistent laxity and high graft failure rates. Zhao et al. evaluated the outcomes of PCL reconstruction augmented with an internal brace system.

The authors present a retrospective analysis of patients treated for isolated or combined grade III PCL injuries. They exclusively included those who underwent PCL reconstruction using hamstring tendon autografts augmented with high-strength suture tape via a transtibial tunnel technique. The surgical procedure involved multiple steps to ensure accurate graft placement and secure fixation, aiming to enhance the biomechanical properties of the reconstructed ligament. The study's exclusion criteria were stringent, ensuring a focused patient cohort. Postoperative rehabilitation protocols varied depending on the complexity of the surgery but were designed to protect the reconstructed ligament while promoting recovery of function.

The study represents a significant advance in PCL reconstruction techniques, demonstrating improved posterior stability and subjective knee function in patients at a minimum 2-year follow-up. The use of internal brace augmentation appears to offer additional support during the critical healing phase post-surgery, potentially reducing the need for revision procedures as evidenced by no patient requiring PCL revision surgery during the follow-up period. While promising, the authors acknowledge limitations such as the retrospective nature of the study and heterogeneity among patient injuries. Future research with larger randomized controlled trials is necessary to confirm these findings and further refine treatment strategies for complex PCL injuries.

Bibliography

1. Kim YM, Lee CA, Matava MJ. Clinical results of arthroscopic single-bundle transtibial posterior cruciate ligament reconstruction: a systematic review. Am J Sports Med. 2011;39(2):425–34.
2. Trickey EL. Injuries to the posterior cruciate ligament: diagnosis and treatment of early injuries and reconstruc tion of late instability. Clin Orthop Relat Res. 1980;147:76–81.
3. Zhao J, He Y, Wang J. Arthroscopic treatment of acute tibial avulsion fracture of the posterior cruciate ligament with sutu re fixation technique through Y-shaped bone tunnels. Arthroscopy. 2006;22(2):172–81.
4. Keller PM, Shelbourne KD, McCarroll JR, Rettig AC. Nonoperatively treated isolated posterior cruciate ligament injuries. Am J Sports Med. 1993;21(1):132–6.
5. Gui J, Wang L, Jiang Y, Wang Q, Yu Z, Gu Q. Single-tunnel suture fixation of posterior cruciate ligament avulsion fracture. Arthroscopy: the journal of Arthroscopic & Related. Surgery. 2009;25(1):78–85.
6. Sabat D, Jain A, Kumar V. Displaced posterior cruciate ligament avulsion fractures: a retrospective comparative study between open posterior approach and arthroscopic single-tunnel suture fixation. Arthroscopy. 2016;32(1):44–53.
7. Cooper DE, Warren RF, Warner JJP. The posterior cruciate ligament and posterolateral structures of the knee anatomy, functions and pattern of injury. Instr Course Lect. 1991;40:249–70.
8. Fanelli GC, Beck JD, Edson CJ. Current concepts review: the posterior cruciate ligament. J Knee Surg. 2010;23(2):61–72.
9. Houe T, Jorgensen U. Arthroscopic posterior cruciate ligament reconstruction: one- vs. two-tunnel technique. Scand J Med Sci Sports. 2004;14:107–11.
10. Wang CJ, Weng LH, Hsu CC, Chan YS. Arthroscopic single versus double-bundle posterior cruciate ligament reconstructions using hamstring autograft. Injury. 2004;35:1293–9.
11. Deie M, Adachi N, Nakamae A, Takazawa K, Ochi M. Evaluation of single-bundle versus double-bundle PCL reconstructions with more than 10-year follow up. Sci World J. 2015;2015:751465.
12. Schulz MS, Russe K, Weiler A, Eichhorn HJ, Strobel MJ. Epidemiology of posterior cruciate ligament injuries. Arch Orthop Trauma Surg. 2003;123(4):186–91.
13. Hammoud S, Reinhardt KR, Marx RG. Outcomes of posterior cruciate ligament treatment: a review of the evidence. Sports Med Arthrosc. 2010;18(4):280–91.

14. Kim SJ, Jung M, Moon HK, Kim SG, Chun YM. Anterolateral transtibial posterior cruciate ligament reconstruction combined with anatomical reconstruction of posterolateral corner insufficiency: comparison of single-bundle versus double-bundle posterior cruciate ligament reconstruction over a 2- to 6-year follow-up. Am J Sports Med. 2011;39(3):481–9.
15. Cooper DE, Stewart D. Posterior cruciate ligament reconstruction using single-bundle patella tendon graft with tibial inlay fixation: 2- to 10-year follow-up. Am J Sports Med. 2004;32(2):346–60.
16. Shen G, Xu Y, Dong Q, et al. Arthroscopic posterior cruciate ligament reconstruction using LARS artificial ligament: a retrospective study. J Surg Res. 2012;173(1):75–82.
17. Shino K, Horibe S, Nakata K, et al. Conservative treatment of isolated injuries to the posterior cruciate ligament in athletes. J Bone Joint Surg Br. 1995;77:895–900.
18. Chen B, Gao S. Double-bundle posterior cruciate ligament reconstruction using a non-hardware suspension fixation technique and 8 strands of autogenous hamstring tendons. Arthroscopy. 2009;25(7):777–82.
19. Kim SJ, Kim TE, Jo SB, Kung YP. Comparison of the clinical results of three posterior cruciate ligament reconstruction techniques. J Bone Joint Surg Am. 2009;91(11):2543–9.
20. Deehan DJ, Salmon LJ, Russell VJ, Pinczewski LA. Endoscopic single-bundle posterior cruciate ligament reconstruction: results at minimum 2-year follow-up. Arthroscopy. 2003;19(9):955–62.
21. Chen CH, Chen WJ, Shih CH. Arthroscopic reconstruction of the posterior cruciate ligament: a comparison of quadriceps tendon autograft and quadruple hamstring tendon graft. Arthroscopy. 2002;18:603–12.
22. Shino K, Nakagawa S, Nakamura N, Matsumoto N, Toritsuka Y, Natsu-ume T. Arthroscopic posterior cruciate ligament reconstruction using hamstring tendons: one-incision technique with Endobutton. Arthroscopy. 1996;12(5):638–42.
23. Pinczewski LA, Thuresson P, Otto D, Nyquist F. Arthroscopic posterior cruciate ligament reconstruction using four-strand hamstring tendon graft and interference screws. Arthroscopy. 1997;13(5):661–5.
24. Höher J, Scheffler S, Weiler A. Graft choice and graft fixation in PCL reconstruction. Knee Surg Sports Traumatol Arthrosc. 2003;11(5):297–306.
25. Seon JK, Song EK. Reconstruction of isolated posterior cruciate ligament injuries: a clinical comparison of the transtibial and tibial inlay techniques. Arthroscopy. 2006;22:27–32.
26. Corry IS, Webb JM, Clingeleffer AJ, et al. Arthroscopic reconstruction of the anterior cruciate ligament: a comparison of patellar tendon autograft and four-strand hamstring tendon autograft. Am J Sports Med. 1999;27:444–54.
27. Freedman KB, D'Amato MJ, Nedeff DD, et al. Arthroscopic anterior cruciate ligament reconstruction: a metaanalysis comparing patellar tendon and hamstring tendon autografts. Am J Sports Med. 2003;31:2–11.
28. Pinczewski LA, Lyman J, Salmon LJ, et al. A 10-year comparison of anterior cruciate ligament reconstructions with hamstring tendon and patellar tendon autograft: a controlled, prospective trial. Am J Sports Med. 2007;35:564–74.
29. LaPrade CM, Civitarese DM, Rasmussen MT, LaPrade RF. Emerging updates on the posterior cruciate ligament: a review of the current literature. Am J Sports Med. 2015;43(12):3077–92. (Leading review of current literature on PCL reconstruction).
30. Jackman T, LaPrade RF, Pontinen T, Lender PA. Intraobserver and interobserver reliability of the kneeling technique of stress radiography for the evaluation of posterior knee laxity. Am J Sports Med. 2008;36(8):1571–6. (Introduction of validated imaging method for objective quantification of PCL laxity).
31. Chahla J, Nitri M, Civitarese D, Dean CS, Moulton SG, LaPrade RF. Anatomic double-bundle posterior cruciate ligament reconstruction. Arthrosc Tech. 2016;5(1):e149–56.
32. Sekiya JK, Whiddon DR, Zehms CT, Miller MD. A clinically relevant assessment of posterior cruciate ligament and posterolateral corner injuries. Evaluation of isolated and combined

deficiency. J Bone Joint Surg Am. 2008;90(8):1621–7, A Clinically Relevant Assessment of Posterior Cruciate Ligament and Posterolateral Corner Injuries.
33. Bergfeld JA, Graham SM, Parker RD, Valdevit AD, Kambic HE. A biomechanical comparison of posterior cruciate ligament reconstructions using single- and double-bundle tibial inlay techniques. Am J Sports Med. 2005;33(7):976–81.
34. Harner CD, Janaushek MA, Kanamori A, Yagi M, Vogrin TM, Woo SL. Biomechanical analysis of a double-bundle posterior cruciate ligament reconstruction. Am J Sports Med. 2000;28(2):144–51.
35. Mannor DA, Shearn JT, Grood ES, Noyes FR, Levy MS. Two-bundle posterior cruciate ligament reconstruction. An in vitro analysis of graft placement and tension. Am J Sports Med. 2000;28(6):833–45.
36. Milles JL, Nuelle CW, Pfeiffer F, Stannard JP, Smith P, Kfuri M Jr, et al. Biomechanical comparison: single-bundle versus double-bundle posterior cruciate ligament reconstruction techniques. J Knee Surg. 2017;30(4):347–51.
37. Wijdicks CA, Kennedy NI, Goldsmith MT, Devitt BM, Michalski MP, Årøen A, et al. Kinematic analysis of the posterior cruciate ligament, part 2: a comparison of anatomic single- versus double-bundle reconstruction. Am J Sports Med. 2013;41(12):2839–48.
38. Lee DY. Single-bundle versus double-bundle posterior cruciate ligament reconstruction: a meta-analysis of randomized controlled. Trials. 2017;29(4):246–55.
39. Carson EW, Deng XH, Allen A, Wickiewicz T, Warren RF. Evaluation of in situ graft forces of a 2-bundle tibial inlay posterior cruciate ligament reconstruction at various flexion angles. Arthroscopy. 2007;23(5):488–95.
40. Matava MJ, Ellis E, Gruber B. Surgical treatment of posterior cruciate ligament tears: an evolving technique. J Am Acad Orthop Surg. 2009;17(7):435–46.
41. Makino A, Costa-Paz M, Aponte-Tinao L, Ayerza MA, Muscolo DL. Popliteal artery laceration during arthroscopic posterior cruciate ligament reconstruction. Arthroscopy. 2005;21(11):1396.
42. Wu RW, Hsu CC, Wang CJ. Acute popliteal artery occlusion after arthroscopic posterior cruciate ligament reconstruction. Arthroscopy. 2003;19(8):889–93.
43. Zawodny SR, Miller MD. Complications of posterior cruciate ligament surgery. Sports Med Arthrosc Rev. 2010;18(4):269–74.
44. Noyes FR, Barber-Westin SD. Posterior cruciate ligament revision reconstruction, part 1: causes of surgical failure in 52 consecutive operations. Am J Sports Med. 2005;33(5):646–54.
45. Belk JW, Kraeutler MJ, Purcell JM, McCarty EC. Autograft versus allograft for posterior cruciate ligament reconstruction: an updated systematic review and meta-analysis. Am J Sports Med. 2017;46:1752–7. https://doi.org/10.1177/0363546517713164.
46. Park HG, Ham HJ. Effect of posteromedial corner injury on stability and second-look arthroscopic findings after posterior cruciate ligament reconstruction using allograft. J Orthop. 2020;22:104–8.
47. Tian P, Hu WQ, Li ZJ, Sun XL, Ma XL. Comparison of autograft and allograft tendons in posterior cruciate ligament reconstruction: a meta-analysis. Medicine (Baltimore). 2017;96:e7434.
48. Ahn JH, Yoo JC, Wang JH. Posterior cruciate ligament reconstruction: double-loop hamstring tendon autograft versus Achilles tendon allograft–clinical results of a minimum 2-year follow-up. Arthroscopy. 2005;21:965–9.
49. Kim SJ, Kim HK, Kim HJ. Arthroscopic posterior cruciate ligament reconstruction using a one-incision technique. Clin Orthop Relat Res. 1999;359:156–66. https://doi.org/10.1097/00003086-199902000-00017156-166.
50. Li B, Wang JS, He M, et al. Comparison of hamstring tendon autograft and tibialis anterior allograft in arthroscopic transtibial single-bundle posterior cruciate ligament reconstruction. Knee Surg Sports Traumatol Arthrosc. 2015;23(10):3077–84.
51. Sun X, Zhang J, Qu X, Zheng Y. Arthroscopic posterior cruciate ligament reconstruction with allograft versus autograft. Arch Med Sci. 2015;11:395–401.

52. Wang CJ, Chan YS, Weng LH, Yuan LJ, Chen HS. Comparison of autogenous and allogenous posterior cruciate ligament reconstructions of the knee. Injury. 2004;35(12):1279–85.
53. Xu M, Zhang Q, Dai S, Teng X, Liu Y, Ma Z. Double bundle versus single bundle reconstruction in the treatment of posterior cruciate ligament injury: a prospective comparative study. Indian J Orthop. 2019;53:297–303.
54. Setyawan R, Soekarno NR, Asikin AIZ, Rhatomy S. Posterior cruciate ligament reconstruction with peroneus longus tendon graft: 2-years follow-up. Ann Med Surg (Lond). 2019;43:38–43.
55. Kang SH, Sohn KM, Lee DK, Lee BH, Yang SW, Wang JH. Arthroscopic posterior cruciate ligament reconstruction: the achilles tendon allograft versus the quadriceps tendon allograft. J Knee Surg. 2020;33:553–9.
56. Forsythe B, Haro MS, Bogunovic L, Collins MJ, Arns TA, Trella KJ, et al. Biomechanical evaluation of posterior cruciate ligament reconstruction with quadriceps versus achilles tendon bone block allograft. Orthop J Sports Med. 2016;4:2325967116660068.
57. Dericks G Jr. Ligament advanced reinforcement system anterior cruciate ligament reconstruction. Oper Tech Sports Med. 1995;3:187–205.
58. Brunet P, Charrois O, Degeorges R, Boisrenoult P, Beaufils P. Reconstruction of acute posterior cruciate ligament tears using a synthetic ligament (in French). Rev Chir Orthop Reparatrice Appar Mot. 2005;91:34–43.
59. Crossley KM, Bennell KL, Cowan SM, Green S. Analysis of outcome measures for persons with patellofemoral pain: which are reliable and valid? Arch Phys Med Rehabil. 2004;85:815–22.
60. Chahla J, Moatshe G, Cinque ME, Dornan GJ, Mitchell JJ, Ridley TJ, et al. Single-bundle and double-bundle posterior cruciate ligament reconstructions: a systematic review and meta-analysis of 441 patients at a minimum 2 years' follow-up. Arthroscopy. 2017;33:2066–80.
61. Heusdens CHW, Hopper GP, Dossche L, Roelant E, Mackay GM. Anterior cruciate ligament repair with independent suture tape reinforcement: a case series with 2-year follow-up. Knee Surg Sports TraumatolArthrosc. 2019;27:60–7.
62. Spindler KP, Huston LJ, Wright RW, Kaeding CC, Marx RG, Amendola A, et al. The prognosis and predictors of sports function and activity at minimum 6 years after anterior cruciate ligament reconstruction: a population cohort study. Am J Sports Med. 2011;39:348–59.
63. Wheatley WB, Martinez AE, Sacks T, Schurhoff MR, Uribe JW, Hechtman KS, et al. Arthroscopic posterior cruciate ligament repair. Arthroscopy. 2002;18:695–702.
64. Grotting JA, Nelson TJ, Banffy MB, et al. Biomechanical evaluation of PCL reconstruction with suture augmentation. Knee. 2020;27:375–83.
65. Trasolini NA, Hatch GF, Wright D, Levy BA, Stuart MJ, McGarry MH, Lee TQ. Posterior cruciate ligament reconstruction with internal brace augmentation reduces posterior tibial translation under cyclic loading. Orthopedics. 2021;44(4):235–40.
66. Lai VJ, Reynolds AW, Kindya M, Konicek J, Akhavan S. The use of suture augmentation for graft protection in ACL reconstruction: a biomechanical study in porcine knees. Arthrosc Sports Med Rehabil. 2020;3(1):e57–63.
67. van der List JP, DiFelice GS. Arthroscopic primary posterior cruciate ligament repair with suture augmentation. Arthrosc Tech. 2017;6(5):e1685–90.
68. Xu Z, Dong Y, Feng Y-e, Xie P, Gu J, Kang K, Gao S, Zheng X. A simple arthroscopic technique for treatment of displaced "hinged" type of posterior cruciate ligament avulsion fractures. BMC Musculoskelet Disord. 2022;23:841. https://doi.org/10.1186/s12891-022-05795-8.
69. Luo Y, Wang Z-g, Li Z-j, Wei M. Arthroscopic reconstruction of the posterior cruciate ligament with a ligament-advanced reinforcement system and hamstring tendon autograft: a retrospective study. Curr Med Sci. 2021;41:930–5. https://doi.org/10.1007/s11596-021-2446-7.
70. Jain V, Goyal A, Mohindra M, Kumar R, Joshi D, Chaudhary D. A comparative analysis of arthroscopic double-bundle versus single-bundle posterior cruciate ligament reconstruction using hamstring tendon autograft. Arch Orthop Trauma Surg. 2016;136:1555–61. https://doi.org/10.1007/s00402-016-2512-y.

71. Boutefnouchet T, Bentayeb M, Qadri Q, Ali S. Long-term outcomes following single-bundle transtibial arthroscopic posterior cruciate ligament reconstruction. Int Orthop. 2012;37:337–43. https://doi.org/10.1007/s00264-012-1609-3.
72. Xu X, Huang T, Liu Z, Wen H, Ye L, Hu Y, Yu H, Pan X. Hamstring tendon autograft versus LARS artificial ligament for arthroscopic posterior cruciate ligament reconstruction in a long-term follow-up. Arch Orthop Trauma Surg. 2014;134:1753–9. https://doi.org/10.1007/s00402-014-2104-7.
73. Norbakhsh ST, Zafarani Z, Najafi A, Aslani H. Arthroscopic posterior cruciate ligament reconstruction by using hamstring tendon autograft and transosseous screw fixation: minimal 3 years follow-up. Arch Orthop Trauma Surg. 2014;134:1723–30. https://doi.org/10.1007/s00402-014-2082-9.
74. Lin Y-C, Chen S-K, Liu T-H, Cheng Y-M, Chou PP-H. Arthroscopic transtibial single-bundle posterior cruciate ligament reconstruction using patellar tendon graft compared with hamstring tendon graft. Arch Orthop Trauma Surg. 2013;133:523–30. https://doi.org/10.1007/s00402-013-1679-8.
75. Johnson P, Mitchell SM, Görtz S. Graft considerations in posterior cruciate ligament reconstruction. Curr Rev Musculoskelet Med. 2018;11:521–7. https://doi.org/10.1007/s12178-018-9506-z.
76. Migliorini F, Pintore A, Oliva F, Eschweiler J, Bell A, Maffulli N. Allografts as alternative to autografts in primary posterior cruciate ligament reconstruction: a systematic review and meta-analysis. Knee Surg Sports Traumatol Arthrosc. 2022;30:1282–91. https://doi.org/10.1007/s00167-022-07258-y.
77. Li B, Wen Y, Wu H, Qian Q, Wu Y, Lin X. Arthroscopic single-bundle posterior cruciate ligament reconstruction: retrospective review of hamstring tendon graft versus LARS artificial ligament. Int Orthop. 2008;33:991–6. https://doi.org/10.1007/s00264-008-0628-6.
78. Hopper GP, Irfan A, Jenkins JM, Wilson WT, Mackay GM. Posterior cruciate ligament repair with suture tape augmentation: a case series with minimum 2-year follow-up. J Exp Orthop. 2021;8:28. https://doi.org/10.1186/s40634-021-00337-y.
79. Zhao X, Duan MY, Chen SQ, Wang J, Li W, Lv Y, Zhang HZ. Posterior cruciate ligament reconstruction with independent internal brace reinforcement: surgical technique and clinical outcomes with a minimum two year follow-up. Int Orthop. 2022;46:2019–28. https://doi.org/10.1007/s00264-022-05448-4.

Chapter 15
Medial Collateral Ligament Tears

Alfred J. Tria Jr. and Giles R. Scuderi

Machine Generated Summaries

Disclaimer: The summaries in this chapter were generated from Springer Nature publications using abstractive AI auto-summarization: An abstraction-based summarizer creates new text based on deep learning. New phrases are created to summarize the content. As the constituted sentences are machine selected, they may not fully reflect the body of the work, so we strongly advise that the original content is read and cited. The auto-generated summaries were curated by the editor to meet Springer Nature publication standards.

Machine generated keywords: smcl, brace, construct, length, internal brace, mcl reconstruction, allograft, internal, mcl internal, stability, early, intact, load, loading, mcl plus

Limited Surgical Techniques

Machine generated keywords: brace, construct, internal brace, internal, mcl internal, intact, ligament brace, mcl ligament, reveal, cyclic, construct specimen, lesion, deflection, fatigue, acl replacement

A. J. Tria Jr. (✉)
Department of Orthopedics, Rutgers-Robert Wood Johnson Medical School, New Brunswick, NJ, USA

G. R. Scuderi
Northwell Health Orthopaedic Institute, New York, NY, USA

A. J. Tria Jr., G. R. Scuderi (eds.), *Ligaments of the Knee*,
https://doi.org/10.1007/978-3-031-66615-5_15

MCL Internal Brace Does Not Fully Recapitulate Normal MCL Function in Valgus Stress [76]

This is a machine-generated summary of:

Tompkins, Marc A.; Freeman, Andrew L.; Hursh, Elliot; Bechtold, Joan E.: MCL internal brace does not fully recapitulate normal MCL function in valgus stress [76]

Published in: Knee Surgery, Sports Traumatology, Arthroscopy (2023)

Link to original: https://doi.org/10.1007/s00167-023-07438-4

If you want to cite the papers, please refer to the original.

For technical reasons we could not place the page where the original quote is coming from.

Research Highlights

The medial collateral ligament (MCL) is a critical structure for knee stability, particularly against valgus forces. Despite its robustness, MCL injuries are common in sports, leading to significant downtime for athletes. While conservative management is often the first line of treatment, surgical intervention may be necessary when conservative measures fail or in cases of multi-ligament injuries. Tompkins aet al.address the biomechanical efficacy of a minimally invasive MCL internal brace technique under valgus stress testing.

Tompkins utilized cadaveric specimens to simulate MCL injuries and repair using two different internal brace constructs. They prepared eight matched pairs of cadaver knees, ensuring that each knee was free from pre-existing ligament damage and only exhibited mild degenerative changes. They then proceeded with the surgical application of the internal brace constructs, employing techniques to replicate clinical scenarios as closely as possible. Their goal was to evaluate these constructs in a way that would closely mirror their use in patients.

They applied consistent valgus forces to each knee and used radiographic imaging to measure medial joint space opening, comparing the results between intact MCLs and those with internal braces simulating various grades of injury. The first construct showed no significant difference in maintaining tension during testing compared to intact knees, while the second construct demonstrated improved tension retention but did not fully restore valgus opening to the intact state.

Their findings suggest that while Construct II shows promise in maintaining tension under valgus stress, it does not replicate the native function of an intact

MCL. This insight is vital for clinicians considering this procedure and underscores the need for further clinical studies to assess long-term outcomes and potential benefits in facilitating earlier return to activity post-injury.

Acute MCL and ACL Injuries: First Results of Minimal-Invasive MCL Ligament Bracing with Combined ACL Single-Bundle Reconstruction [77]

This is a machine-generated summary of:

Ateschrang, A.; Döbele, S.; Freude, T.; Stöckle, U.; Schröter, S.; Kraus, T. M.: Acute MCL and ACL injuries: first results of minimal-invasive MCL ligament bracing with combined ACL single-bundle reconstruction [77]

Published in: Archives of Orthopaedic and Trauma Surgery (2016)

Link to original: https://doi.org/10.1007/s00402-016-2497-6

If you want to cite the papers, please refer to the original.

For technical reasons we could not place the page where the original quote is coming from.

Research Highlights

Injuries to the medial collateral ligament (MCL) frequently accompany anterior cruciate ligament (ACL) tears, presenting a complex challenge in orthopedic sports medicine. While the MCL has shown good healing potential, its treatment in conjunction with ACL injuries remains debated, with concerns that improper stability may compromise ACL reconstruction. Ateschrang et al. introduce a novel minimal-invasive technique for MCL bracing combined with ACL reconstruction, aiming to improve postoperative stability and reduce complications such as joint stiffness from arthrofibrosis.

The non-randomized, prospective study involved patients who underwent surgery within days of injury, using a minimal-invasive ligament bracing technique for the MCL and a single-bundle technique for the ACL reconstruction. The authors detailed their methods, from patient selection criteria—acute complete rupture of the ACL with grade II° or III° valgus laxity—to the surgical procedure itself. The MCL stabilization involved securing the ligament with an ultrahigh-molecular-weight polyethylene tape, anchored without extensive soft tissue damage, thus preserving knee structures and potentially reducing recovery complications. Postoperative care followed standardized protocols, and outcomes were measured through various clinical assessments including Lachman test, Rolimeter™ for sagittal stability, and subjective scoring systems like Lysholm and Tegner scores.

The study's main advantage lies in its demonstration that acute combined ACL and MCL lesions can be effectively managed through this new surgical technique, yielding biomechanically stable knees with promising clinical outcomes. Notably, the incidence of postoperative arthrofibrosis was low at 0%, suggesting that this approach may mitigate one of the primary concerns associated with combined ligament surgeries. Their findings contribute insights into the treatment of complex knee injuries, though they acknowledge limitations such as small sample size and lack of a control group. As this is the first trial to describe such a procedure, further research with larger cohorts and longer follow-up periods will be essential to validate these results.

An MCL Internal Brace Can Withstand Cyclic Fatigue Loading and Produce a Valgus Load to Failure Similar to that of Intact Knees [78]

This is a machine-generated summary of:

Tompkins, Marc A.; Williams, Hanna; Bechtold, Joan E.: An MCL internal brace can withstand cyclic fatigue loading and produce a valgus load to failure similar to that of intact knees [78]

Published in: Knee Surgery, Sports Traumatology, Arthroscopy (2023)

Link to original: https://doi.org/10.1007/s00167-023-07439-3

If you want to cite the papers, please refer to the original.

For technical reasons we could not place the page where the original quote is coming from.

Research Highlights

The medial collateral ligament (MCL) is crucial for knee stability, and its injury can be managed conservatively, often without surgery. However, when an MCL injury occurs alongside an anterior cruciate ligament (ACL) tear, treatment becomes more complex due to conflicting rehabilitation needs. Tompkins et al. evaluate the biomechanical durability and strength of a minimally invasive internal brace construct designed to protect the MCL during early healing.

Their research involved biomechanical testing on eight cadaver knee specimens with surgically created Grade III MCL tears. The internal brace construct tested was previously shown to withstand static valgus stress. The current study aimed to assess its performance under cyclic loading conditions that mimic daily activities, using a servo-hydraulic testing machine and a custom MATLAB program for data analysis. They applied a pre-load followed by cyclic loading and a final load-to-failure test to measure the construct's deflection angles, stiffness, and ultimate failure load.

The findings revealed that the internal brace construct maintained tension throughout fatigue testing, with minimal change in deflection angle and an average failure bending moment within the range of an intact MCL. These results suggest that the surgical construct could effectively protect the MCL during the healing process. Despite limitations such as lack of a control group and not accounting for tissue healing responses in living subjects, this study provides valuable insights for clinicians considering this technique for MCL protection.

Primary Surgical Repair

Machine generated keywords: irreducible, group, augmentation, suture tape, tape augmentation, mcl repair, unstable, tape, iii mcl, repair mcl, suture, aclr, suture repair

Suture Tape Augmentation Improves Laxity of MCL Repair in the ACL Reconstructed Knee [79]

This is a machine-generated summary of:

van Eck, Carola F.; Nakamura, Tomomasa; Price, Taylor; Linde, Monica; Smolinski, Patrick: Suture tape augmentation improves laxity of MCL repair in the ACL reconstructed knee [79]

Published in: Knee Surgery, Sports Traumatology, Arthroscopy (2021)

Link to original: https://doi.org/10.1007/s00167-020-06386-7

If you want to cite the papers, please refer to the original.

For technical reasons we could not place the page where the original quote is coming from.

Research Highlights

Suture anchor repair, particularly with internal bracing or suture tape augmentation, has revolutionized the approach to orthopedic surgeries, offering benefits such as reduced surgical times and expedited recovery for athletes. Despite its growing popularity in procedures like anterior cruciate ligament (ACL) and elbow ulnar collateral ligament surgery, the impact of suture tape augmentation on knee kinematics in combined ACL and medial collateral ligament (MCL) injuries remains unexplored van Eck et al. investigate the biomechanical effects of MCL suture repair with and without suture tape augmentation in the setting of concurrent ACL reconstruction (ACLR).

The University of Pittsburgh's Committee for Oversight of Research and Clinical Training Involving Decedents approved this human cadaver study, which utilized fresh-frozen specimens to simulate knee conditions. The researchers employed a six-degrees-of-freedom robotic system to test four loading conditions on knees that were free from significant arthritic changes or anatomic variants that could skew results. The study measured displacement, rotation, and forces within the MCL under various states—intact, suture repaired, and augmented with suture tape—following ACLR using an anatomic technique.

The authors used a suture anchor loaded with suture tape for MCL repair, ensuring precise fixation at specific knee flexion angles. While neither MCL repair alone nor with suture tape augmentation perfectly restored knee kinematics under valgus load to the intact state, the addition of suture tape significantly improved rotational stability.

Their findings suggest that augmenting MCL repair with suture tape can enhance knee stability without causing over-constraint—a concern among surgeons considering this technique. This could lead to better outcomes for patients with combined ACL-MCL injuries by potentially reducing failure rates and residual instability while allowing for more aggressive rehabilitation protocols.

The results are promising but also highlight the need for further research. Future research should focus on clinical trials to validate these findings in vivo and refine surgical techniques and postoperative care accordingly.

Early Medial Reconstruction Combined with Severely Injured Medial Collateral Ligaments Can Decrease Residual Medial Laxity in Anterior Cruciate Ligament Reconstruction [80]

This is a machine-generated summary of:

Sim, Jae Ang; Na, Young Gon; Choi, Ji Wook; Lee, Byung Hoon: Early medial reconstruction combined with severely injured medial collateral ligaments can decrease residual medial laxity in anterior cruciate ligament reconstruction [80]

Published in: Archives of Orthopaedic and Trauma Surgery (2021)

Link to original: https://doi.org/10.1007/s00402-021-04211-5

If you want to cite the papers, please refer to the original.

For technical reasons we could not place the page where the original quote is coming from.

Research Highlights

Anterior cruciate ligament (ACL) injuries often occur in conjunction with medial collateral ligament (MCL) damage, presenting a complex clinical challenge. While isolated ACL reconstructions have shown success, the optimal treatment for combined ACL and grade III MCL injuries, which can lead to chronic valgus instability, remains debated. Sim et al. compare the outcomes of initial MCL reconstruction versus primary MCL repair in patients with combined ACL and grade III MCL injuries, hypothesizing that early graft reconstructions may better prevent chronic instability and facilitate rehabilitation.

In this retrospective study, patients who underwent anatomical ACL reconstruction between 2008 and 2017 were assessed. The authors categorized patients based on the presence and treatment of concomitant MCL injuries. Utilizing magnetic resonance imaging and valgus stress testing under anesthesia, the severity of MCL injuries was determined preoperatively. The surgical procedures were consistently performed by an experienced surgeon at a single institution, ensuring uniformity in technique and postoperative care.

Patients were divided into groups: those with isolated ACL ruptures (Group A) and those with combined ACL and MCL injuries (Group B), with further subdivisions in Group B based on MCL injury severity and treatment modality. The study recorded concomitant meniscal injuries, surgical techniques for both ACL and MCL reconstructions, and postoperative rehabilitation protocols.

Clinical outcomes were evaluated using Lysholm knee scores, Tegner activity levels, and Likert scales for satisfaction measurement. Radiographic measurements provided objective data on valgus laxity over time.

The key finding is that primary medial reconstruction results in less medial opening over time compared to primary repair, although both methods showed similar clinical outcomes at the two-year follow-up. This suggests that while immediate structural stability is crucial, long-term clinical success may not be significantly influenced by the choice between repair or reconstruction of the MCL.

The study also highlights a higher incidence of concomitant meniscal injuries in combined ACL-MCL injuries than in isolated ACL tears, emphasizing the need for careful evaluation during treatment planning. The authors conclude that primary medial reconstruction may offer a more stable solution for severe MCL damage accompanying ACL ruptures.

Secondary Reconstruction

Machine generated keywords: smcl, length, mcl reconstruction, allograft, stability, mcl plus, plus, length change, plus acl, combine mcl, isolated mcl, kinematic stability, graft

Single Allograft Medial Collateral Ligament and Posterior Oblique Ligament Reconstruction: A Technique to Improve Valgus and Rotational Stability [81]

This is a machine-generated summary of:

Dong, Jiangtao; Ji, Gang; Zhang, Yingze; Gao, Shijun; Wang, Fei; Chen, Baicheng: Single allograft medial collateral ligament and posterior oblique ligament reconstruction: a technique to improve valgus and rotational stability [81]

Published in: European Journal of Orthopaedic Surgery & Traumatology (2013)

Link to original: https://doi.org/10.1007/s00590-013-1265-3

If you want to cite the papers, please refer to the original.

For technical reasons we could not place the page where the original quote is coming from.

Research Highlights

The medial collateral ligament (MCL) is a key component in maintaining knee stability, with its integrity being essential for preventing valgus and rotational stresses. Despite advances in surgical techniques, restoring both valgus and rotational stability remains a challenge. Dong et al. present a surgical procedure aimed at repairing the MCL to address both types of instability simultaneously.

They developed a method that involves reconstructing the MCL and the posterior oblique ligament (POL) using a double-bundle technique with allografts. This approach creates a triangular functional area that enhances stability by leveraging the anatomical positioning of femoral and tibial insertions. The surgery begins with careful arthroscopic evaluations to assess intra-articular damage and MCL injury, followed by preparation of allografts and bone tunnels. The grafts are then strategically placed and fixed, ensuring restoration of stability without compromising the knee's dynamic structures such as the semimembranosus and pes anserinus. Postoperative treatment includes targeted rehabilitation to promote healing while maintaining strength and flexibility.

The technique addresses both valgus and rotational instabilities, which traditional methods often fail to achieve simultaneously. By using allografts instead of autografts, the procedure also minimizes potential damage to dynamic stabilizers.

The Superficial Medial Collateral Ligament Reconstruction of the Knee: Effect of Altering Graft Length on Knee Kinematics and Stability [82]

This is a machine-generated summary of:

Van den Bogaerde, J. M.; Shin, E.; Neu, C. P.; Marder, R. A.: The superficial medial collateral ligament reconstruction of the knee: effect of altering graft length on knee kinematics and stability [82]

Published in: Knee Surgery, Sports Traumatology, Arthroscopy (2011)

Link to original: https://doi.org/10.1007/s00167-011-1519-8

If you want to cite the papers, please refer to the original.

For technical reasons we could not place the page where the original quote is coming from.

Research Highlights

Injuries to the medial collateral ligament (MCL) of the knee, particularly when combined with damage to other ligaments, can lead to chronic instability. While isolated MCL injuries often heal without surgery, more complex cases involving the superficial MCL (sMCL) and posterior oblique ligament (POL) may require reconstruction to prevent persistent valgus laxity. den Bogaerde et al. investigate the biomechanical effects of sMCL reconstruction using grafts of different lengths on knee kinematics and stability.

The authors utilized 12 human cadaver leg specimens to simulate active knee extension and passive joint stability testing. They hypothesized that using hamstring tendon grafts matching the normal sMCL length would best restore natural knee function. An electromagnetic tracking device measured knee movements during testing, ensuring precise detection of even minor rotational differences. The study compared intact knees, knees with divided sMCL, and knees reconstructed with two different graft lengths—one matching the native sMCL and another equal to the patellar tendon length.

The authors found that anatomically accurate reconstructions (AnatRecon) closely replicated normal knee kinematics and stability, while shorter grafts (ShortRecon) led to significant deviations in rotational stability during both active extension and passive testing. These findings underscore the importance of restoring the sMCL's anatomic length for successful reconstruction.

This study suggests that anatomical reconstruction of the sMCL is crucial for maintaining normal joint kinematics, as non-anatomic reconstructions can result in altered motion patterns and potential instability. The authors advocate for future clinical trials to evaluate the efficacy of anatomic versus non-anatomic MCL reconstructions in patients, which could lead to improved surgical outcomes for those suffering from severe medial knee injuries.

Medial Collateral Ligament Reconstruction Graft Isometry Is Effected by Femoral Position More than Tibial Position [83]

This is a machine-generated summary of:

Kittl, Christoph; Robinson, James; Raschke, Michael J.; Olbrich, Arne; Frank, Andre; Glasbrenner, Johannes; Herbst, Elmar; Domnick, Christoph; Herbort, Mirco: Medial collateral ligament reconstruction graft isometry is effected by femoral position more than tibial position [83]

Published in: Knee Surgery, Sports Traumatology, Arthroscopy (2021)

Link to original: https://doi.org/10.1007/s00167-020-06420-8

If you want to cite the papers, please refer to the original.

For technical reasons we could not place the page where the original quote is coming from.

Research Highlights

The medial ligament complex, comprising the superficial medial collateral ligament (sMCL) and the posterior oblique ligament (POL), plays a crucial role in maintaining knee stability. While most minor MCL injuries can be treated non-surgically, more severe or combined injuries often lead to persistent instability and may require reconstruction. However, achieving biomechanical fidelity in medial reconstructions remains challenging due to the complex anatomy and behavior of these ligaments. Kittl et al. investigated the length change patterns of native knee structures to inform optimal graft placement in medial reconstructions.

Kittl utilized eight fresh-frozen cadaveric knee specimens to map out the native length change patterns of the sMCL and POL during knee flexion. The authors prepared each specimen, ensuring accurate representation of the medial knee anatomy. They then tested various femoral and tibial attachment points for sMCL and POL reconstructions, using a custom rig to measure changes in ligament length with knee movement. By comparing these patterns with those of native ligaments, they aimed to identify optimal attachment sites that would best replicate natural ligament behavior.

The study revealed that small alterations in femoral attachment sites significantly impacted the length change behavior of medial reconstruction grafts. The most isometric behavior was observed in the middle portion of the MCL, while the POL exhibited more anisometric patterns. Reconstructions that closely mirrored native sMCL length changes were achieved when using the semitendinosus tendon with minimal alteration to its tibial attachment point. These findings suggest that precise placement of grafts is critical for successful medial knee reconstructions.

In conclusion, this research highlights how slight variations in graft placement can substantially affect post-reconstruction outcomes. Their work underscores the importance of the surgical technique in reproducing native ligament function and suggests that surgeons should prioritize femoral attachment positioning during medial reconstructions. The study also supports tensioning POL grafts near full extension to prevent over-constraint or premature graft failure.

Medial Collateral Ligament (MCL) Reconstruction Results in Improved Medial Stability: Results from the Danish Knee Ligament Reconstruction Registry (DKRR) [84]

This is a machine-generated summary of:

Lind, Martin; Jacobsen, Kevin; Nielsen, Torsten: Medial collateral ligament (MCL) reconstruction results in improved medial stability: results from the Danish knee ligament reconstruction registry (DKRR) [84]

Published in: Knee Surgery, Sports Traumatology, Arthroscopy (2019)

Link to original: https://doi.org/10.1007/s00167-019-05535-x

If you want to cite the papers, please refer to the original.

For technical reasons we could not place the page where the original quote is coming from.

Research Highlights

The medial collateral ligament (MCL) is a critical structure for knee stability, frequently injured in sports-related activities. While most MCL injuries are treated non-operatively, severe cases, especially those associated with anterior cruciate ligament (ACL) tears, pose a challenge. Lind et al. investigated the treatment outcomes for isolated MCL reconstructions versus combined MCL and ACL reconstructions using data from the Danish Knee Ligament Reconstruction Registry (DKRR).

Lind conducted a retrospective analysis of patients who underwent isolated ACL, isolated MCL, or combined MCL and ACL reconstructions between 2005 and 2015. The DKRR provided a dataset, with high registration completeness ensured by mandatory reporting in Denmark. The study's methodology was comprehensive, involving pre-operative and intra-operative data collection by surgeons and post-operative self-assessment questionnaires from patients. The primary outcome measures included the Knee Injury and Osteoarthritis Outcome Score (KOOS) and valgus knee stability assessments.

The results revealed that both isolated MCL reconstruction and combined procedures led to significant improvements in subjective outcomes at the one-year follow-up. Interestingly, while combined MCL plus ACL reconstructions showed lower subjective success rates compared to isolated ACL reconstructions, there was no significant difference between isolated MCL reconstructions and combined procedures. These findings suggest that while MCL reconstruction can improve clinical outcomes, the presence of an accompanying ACL injury does not necessarily worsen the prognosis.

This study confirms that isolated MCL reconstruction can yield significant improvements in knee function and quality of life. However, it also highlights that combined MCL plus ACL reconstructions do not result in inferior outcomes compared to isolated ACL repairs. Looking forward, this work underscores the importance of considering individual patient scenarios when deciding on surgical interventions for complex knee injuries.

Short- to Mid-term Outcomes of Anatomic MCL Reconstruction with Achilles Tendon Allograft After Multiligament Knee Injury [85]

This is a machine-generated summary of:

Barrett, Ian J.; Krych, Aaron J.; Pareek, Ayoosh; Johnson, Nicholas R.; Dahm, Diane L.; Stuart, Michael J.; Levy, Bruce A.: Short- to mid-term outcomes of anatomic MCL reconstruction with Achilles tendon allograft after multiligament knee injury [85]

Published in: Knee Surgery, Sports Traumatology, Arthroscopy (2018)

Link to original: https://doi.org/10.1007/s00167-018-4843-4

If you want to cite the papers, please refer to the original.

For technical reasons we could not place the page where the original quote is coming from.

Research Highlights

The medial collateral ligament complex is crucial for knee stability, yet injuries to this structure are common, affecting numerous individuals annually. Despite the complexity of the medial knee anatomy and the variety of treatment strategies, there remains a lack of consensus on optimal management for medial knee injuries. Barrett et al. report on the clinical and functional outcomes of a modified Marx technique for medial collateral ligament (MCL) reconstruction in multiligament knee injury (MLKI) cases.

The research involved a retrospective analysis of 32 knees in patients who underwent MCL reconstruction using an Achilles tendon bone allograft. The study spanned several years and was conducted by a team of sports medicine fellowship-trained surgeons at a single institution. The modified Marx technique included posteromedial capsular repair with soft tissue anchors and suture anchors at the tibial MCL attachment sites. The team followed a standardized post-operative rehabilitation protocol, ensuring consistency across cases.

Patients were selected based on MRI-confirmed complete MCL disruption and clinically significant valgus instability, with most having sustained their injuries through high-energy mechanisms like motor vehicle accidents. The methodology included fluoroscopic stress examination under anesthesia and grading according to LaPrade criteria. The authors defined treatment failure as reoperation for persistent symptomatic valgus instability or asymmetric medial gapping, which was critical for assessing the technique's efficacy.

The modified Marx technique demonstrated promising results in reducing valgus laxity while maintaining range of motion and yielding high subjective outcome scores. Their findings suggest that anatomic MCL reconstruction can be successfully employed in MLKI settings, indicating that even in severe cases, patients can expect satisfactory outcomes. The correlation between knee dislocation grade and post-operative scores offers a predictive framework for clinical improvement.

Bibliography

1. Fetto JF, Marshall JL. Medial collateral ligament injuries of the knee: a rationale for treatment. Clin Orthop Relat Res. 1978;132:206–18.
2. Ma CB, Papageogiou CD, Debski RE, Woo SL. Interaction between the ACL graft and MCL in a combined ACL+MCL knee injury using a goat model. Acta Orthop Scand. 2000;71:387–93.
3. Grant JA, Tannenbaum E, Miller BS, Bedi A. Treatment of combined complete tears of the anterior cruciate and medial collateral ligaments. Arthroscopy. 2012;28:110–22.
4. Halinen J, Lindahl J, Hirvensalo E, Santavirta S. Operative and nonoperative treatments of medial collateral ligament rupture with early anterior cruciate ligament reconstruction: a prospective randomized study. Am J Sports Med. 2006;34:1134–40.
5. Woo SL, Vogrin TM, Abramowitch SD. Healing and repair of ligament injuries in the knee. J Am Acad Orthop Surg. 2000;8:364–72.
6. Black AK, Schlepp C, Zapf M, Reid JB 3rd. Technique for arthroscopically assisted superficial and deep medial collateral ligament-meniscotibial ligament repair with internal brace augmentation. Arthrosc Tech. 2018;7:e1215–9.

7. Dabis J, Wilson A. Repair and augmentation with internal brace in the multiligament injured knee. Clin Sports Med. 2019;38:275–83.
8. Hirahara AM, Mackay G, Andersen WJ. Ultrasound-guided suture tape augmentation and stabilization of the medial collateral ligament. Arthrosc Tech. 2018;7:e205–10.
9. Lubowitz JH, MacKay G, Gilmer B. Knee medial collateral ligament and posteromedial corner anatomic repair with internal bracing. Arthrosc Tech. 2014;3:e505–8.
10. Mhaskar VA, Mahehswari J, Sansanwal M. Femoral Avulsion of the anterior cruciate ligament in a multiligament setting: a unique case. Knee Surg Relat Res. 2019;31:137–42.
11. Trofa DP, Sonnenfeld JJ, Song DJ, Lynch TS. Distal knee medial collateral ligament repair with suture augmentation. Arthrosc Tech. 2018;7:e921–6.
12. van der List JP, DiFelice GS. Primary repair of the medial collateral ligament with internal bracing. Arthrosc Tech. 2017;6:e933–7.
13. Griffith CJ, LaPrade RF, Johansen S, Armitage B, Wijdicks C, Engebretsen L. Medial knee injury: part 1, static function of the individual components of the main medial knee structures. Am J Sports Med. 2009;37:1762–70.
14. Frisch NB, Keller RA, Mueller JKP, Bandi M, Snethen KG. Treatment of medial collateral ligament injury during total knee arthroplasty with internal suture brace augmentation: a cadaveric and biomechanical study. Orthopedics. 2022;45:e269–75.
15. Duncan JB, Hunter R, Purnell M, Freeman J. Meniscal injuries associated with acute anterior cruciate ligament tears in alpine skiers. Am J Sports Med. 1995;23(2):170–2.
16. Zaffagnini S, Bignozzi S, Martelli S, Lopomo N, Marcacci M. Does ACL reconstruction restore knee stability in combined lesions?: an in vivo study. Clin Orthop Relat Res. 2007;454:95–9.
17. Abramowitch SD, Yagi M, Tsuda E, Woo SL-Y. The healing medial collateral ligament following a combined anterior cruciate and medial collateral ligament injury—a biomechanical study in a goat model. J Orthop Res. 2003;21:1124–30.
18. Kanamori A, Sakane M, Zeminski J, Rudy TW, Woo SL. In-situ force in the medial and lateral structures of intact and ACL-deficient knees. J Orthop Sci. 2000;5(6):567–71.
19. Sakane M, Livesay GA, Fox RJ, Rudy TW, Runco TJ, Woo SL. Relative contribution of the ACL, MCL, and bony contact to the anterior stability of the knee. Knee Surg Sports Traumatol Arthrosc. 1999;7(2):93–7.
20. Yoshiya S, Kuroda R, Mizuno K, Yamamoto T, Kurosaka M. Medial collateral ligament reconstruction using autogenous hamstring tendons: technique and results in initial cases. Am J Sports Med. 2005;33(9):1380–5.
21. Zaffagnini S, Bonanzinga T, Marcheggiani Muccioli GM, Giordano G, Bruni D, Bignozzi S, Lopomo N, Marcacci M. Does chronic medial collateral ligament laxity influence the outcome of anterior cruciate ligament reconstruction?: a prospective evaluation with a minimum three-year follow-up. J Bone Joint Surg Br. 2011;93(8):1060–4.
22. Ibrahim SA. Primary repair of the cruciate and collateral ligaments after traumatic dislocation of the knee. J Bone Joint Surg Br. 1999;81(6):987–90.
23. Owens BD, Neault M, Benson E, Busconi BD. Primary repair of knee dislocations: results in 25 patients (28 knees) at a mean follow-up of four years. J Orthop Trauma. 2007;21(2):92–6.
24. Yeh WL, Tu YK, Su JY, Hsu RW. Knee dislocation: treatment of high-velocity knee dislocation. J Trauma. 1999;46(4):693–701.
25. Halinen J, Lindahl J, Hirvensalo E. Range of motion and quadriceps muscle power after early surgical treatment of acute combined anterior cruciate and grade-III medial collateral ligament injuries. A prospective randomized study. J Bone Joint Surg Am. 2009;91:1305–12.
26. Azar FM. Evaluation and treatment of chronic medial collateral ligament injuries of the knee. Sports Med Arthrosc Rev. 2006;14:84–90.
27. Edson CJ. Conservative and postoperative rehabilitation of isolated and combined injuries of the medial collateral ligament. Sports Med Arthrosc Rev. 2006;14:105–10.
28. Giannotti BF, Rudy T, Graziano J. The non-surgical management of isolated medial collateral ligament injuries of the knee. Sports Med Arthrosc Rev. 2006;14:74–7.

29. Bose D, Bhalla KS, Untaroiu CD, Ivarsson BJ, Crandall JR, Hurwitz S. Injury tolerance and moment response of the knee joint to combined valgus bending and shear loading. J Biomech Eng. 2008;130:031008.
30. Kajzer J, Matsui Y, Ishikawa H, Schroeder G, Bosch U. Shearing and bending effects at the knee joint at low speed lateral loading. SAE Int Tech Pap 1999-01-0712:1–14; 1999.
31. Ramet M, Bouquet R, Bermond F, Caire Y, Bouallegue M. Shearing and bending human knee joint tests in quasi-static lateral load. Paper presented at: proceedings of the international IRCOBI conference on the biomechanics of impact; September 1995; Brunnen, Switzerland; 1995.
32. Gilmer BB, Crall T, DeLong J, Kubo T, Mackay G, Jani SS. Biomechanical analysis of internal bracing for treatment of medial knee injuries. Orthopedics. 2016;39:e532–7.
33. Kanamori A, Zeminski J, Rudy TW, Li G, Fu FH, Woo SL. The effect of axial tibial torque on the function of the anterior cruciate ligament: a biomechanical study of a simulated pivot shift test. Arthroscopy. 2002;18(4):394–8.
34. Kato Y, Ingham SJ, Kramer S, Smolinski P, Saito A, Fu FH. Effect of tunnel position for anatomic single-bundle ACL reconstruction on knee biomechanics in a porcine model. Knee Surg Sports Traumatol Arthrosc. 2010;18:2–10.
35. Kato Y, Maeyama A, Lertwanich P, Wang JH, Ingham SJ, Kramer S, et al. Biomechanical comparison of different graft positions for single-bundle anterior cruciate ligament reconstruction. Knee Surg Sports Traumatol Arthrosc. 2013;21:816–32.
36. Mao Y, Marshall B, Price T, Linde M, Smolinski P, Fu FH, et al. Notchplasty alters knee biomechanics after anatomic ACL reconstruction. Knee Surg Sports Traumatol Arthrosc. 2020;28:614–21.
37. Tischer T, Ronga M, Tsai A, Ingham SJ, Ekdahl M, Smolinski P, et al. Biomechanics of the goat three bundle anterior cruciate ligament. Knee Surg Sports Traumatol Arthrosc. 2009;17:935–40.
38. Mehl JT, Kia C, Murphy M, Obopilwe E, Cote M, Imhoff FB, et al. Posteromedial ligament repair of the knee with suture tape augmentation: a biomechanical study. Am J Sports Med. 2019;47:2952–9.
39. Pandey V, Khanna V, Madi S, Tripathi A, Acharya K. Clinical outcome of primary medial collateral ligament-posteromedial corner repair with or without staged anterior cruciate ligament reconstruction. Injury. 2017;48:1236–42.
40. Harner CD, Irrgang JJ, Paul J, Dearwater S, Fu FH. Loss of motion after anterior cruciate ligament reconstruction. Am J Sports Med. 1992;20:499–506.
41. Noyes FR, Mangine RE, Barber SD. The early treatment of motion complications after reconstruction of the anterior cruciate ligament. Clin Orthop Relat Res. 1992. https://doi.org/10.1097/00003086-199204000-00027.
42. Petersen W, Laprell H. Combined injuries of the medial collateral ligament and the anterior cruciate ligament. Early ACL reconstruction versus late ACL reconstruction. Arch Orthop Trauma Surg. 1999;119(5–6):258–62.
43. Gallo RA, Kozlansky G, Bonazza N, Warren RF. Combined anterior cruciate ligament and medial collateral ligament reconstruction using a single achilles tendon allograft. Arthrosc Tech. 2017;6:e1821–7.
44. Laprade RF, Bernhardson AS, Griffith CJ, Macalena JA, Wijdicks CA. Correlation of valgus stress radiographs with medial knee ligament injuries: an in vitro biomechanical study. Am J Sports Med. 2010;38:330–8.
45. Hillard-Sembell D, Daniel DM, Stone ML, Dobson BE, Fithian DC. Combined injuries of the anterior cruciate and medial collateral ligaments of the knee. Effect of treatment on stability and function of the joint. J Bone Jt Surg Am. 1996;78:169–76.
46. Shelbourne KD, Porter DA. Anterior cruciate ligament-medial collateral ligament injury: nonoperative management of medial collateral ligament tears with anterior cruciate ligament reconstruction. A preliminary report. Am J Sports Med. 1992;20(3):283–6.

47. DeLong JM, Waterman BR. Surgical techniques for the reconstruction of medial collateral ligament and posteromedial corner injuries of the knee: a systematic review. Arthroscopy. 2015. https://doi.org/10.1016/j.arthro.2015.05.011.
48. Moatshe G, Vap AR, Getgood A, LaPrade RF, Engebretsen L. Medial-sided injuries in the multiple ligament knee injury. J Knee Surg. 2020;33:431–9.
49. Hughston JC, Andrews JR, Cross MJ, Moschi A. Classification of knee ligament instabilities. Part I. The medial compartment and cruciate ligaments. J Bone Joint Surg Am. 1976;58:159–72.
50. Robinson JR, Smigielski R, Brown HB Jr. Clinically relevant anatomy of the medial side and posteromedial corner of the knee. In: LaPrade RF, Chahla J, editors. The medial collateral ligament and the posteromedial corner: a comprehensive analysis. New York: Nova Science Publishers, Incorporated; 2018. p. 1–44.
51. Warren LF, Marshall J. The supporting structures and layers on the medial side of the knee: an anatomical analysis. J Bone Joint Surg Am. 1979;61:56–62.
52. Mazzocca AD, Nissen CW, Geary M, Adams DJ. Valgus medial collateral ligament rupture causes concomitant loading and damage of the anterior cruciate ligament. J Knee Surg. 2003;16:148–51.
53. Brantigan OC, Voshell AF. The tibial collateral ligament: its function, its bursae, and its relation to the medial meniscus. J Bone Joint Surg Am. 1943;25:121–31.
54. Hughston JC, Eilers AF. The role of the posterior oblique ligament in repairs of acute medial (collateral) ligament tears of the knee. J Bone Joint Surg Am. 1973;55:923–40.
55. Last R. Some anatomical details of the knee joint. J Bone Joint Surg Br. 1948;30:683–8.
56. LaPrade RF, Engebretsen AH, Ly TV, Johansen S, Wentorf FA, Engebretsen L. The anatomy of the medial part of the knee. J Bone Joint Surg Am. 2007;89:2000–10.
57. Wijdicks CA, Michalski MP, Rasmussen MT, Goldsmith MT, Kennedy NI, Lind M, Engebretsen L, LaPrade RF. Superficial medial collateral ligament anatomic augmented repair versus anatomic reconstruction: an in vitro biomechanical analysis. Am J Sports Med. 2013;41:2858–66.
58. Chen LC, Cooley VJ, Rosenberg TD. Medial collateral ligament healing response technique: microperforation. Tech Knee Surg. 2002;1(1):36–42.
59. Papalia R, Osti L, Del Buono A, Denaro V, Maffulli N. Management of combined ACL-MCL tears: a systematic review. Br Med Bull. 2010;93(1):201–15.
60. Stannard JP. Medial and posteromedial instability of the knee: evaluation, treatment, and results. Sports Med Arthrosc Rev. 2010;18(4):263–8.
61. Millett PJ, Pennock AT, Sterett WI, Steadman JR. Early ACL reconstruction in combined ACL-MCL injuries. J Knee Surg. 2004;17(2):94–8.
62. Piatkowski K, Plominski J, Sowinski T, Piekarczyk P, Kwiatkowski K, Golos J. Results of two-stage operative treatment of anteromedial instability of the knee. Ortop Traumatol Rehabil. 2014;16(1):33–45.
63. Roos EM, Toksvig-Larsen S. Knee injury and Osteoarthritis Outcome Score (KOOS)—validation and comparison to the WOMAC in total knee replacement. Health Qual Life Outcomes. 2003;1:17.
64. Tegner Y, Lysholm J. Rating systems in the evaluation of knee ligament injuries. Clin Orthop Relat Res. 1985;198:43–9.
65. Majewski M, Susanne H, Klaus S. Epidemiology of athletic knee injuries: a 10-year study. Knee. 2006;13:184–8.
66. Laprade RF, Wijdicks CA. Surgical technique: development of an anatomic medial knee reconstruction. Clin Orthop Relat Res. 2012;470(3):806–14.
67. Smyth MP, Koh JL. A review of surgical and nonsurgical outcomes of medial knee injuries. Sports Med Arthrosc. 2015;23:e15–22.
68. Wijdicks CA, Griffith CJ, Johansen S, Engebretsen L, LaPrade RF. Injuries to the medial collateral ligament and associated medial structures of the knee. J Bone Jt Surg Am. 2010;92:1266–80.

69. Marx RG, Stump TJ, Jones EC, Wickiewicz TL, Warren RF. Development and evaluation of an activity rating scale for disorders of the knee. Am J Sports Med. 2001;29(2):213–8.
70. Irrgang JJ, Anderson AF, Boland AL, Harner CD, Kurosaka M, Neyret P, Richmond JC, Shelborne KD. Development and validation of the international knee documentation committee subjective knee form. Am J Sports Med. 2001;29:600–13.
71. Roos EM, Roos HP, Lohmander LS, Ekdahl C, Beynnon BD. Knee injury and osteoarthritis outcome score (KOOS)—development of a self-administered outcome measure. J Orthop Sports Phys Ther. 1998;28:88–96.
72. Leiter JRS, Levy BA, Stannard JP, Fanelli GC, Whelan DB, Marx RG, Stuart MJ, Boyd JL, MacDonald PB. Accuracy and reliability of determining the isometric point of the knee for multiligament knee reconstruction. Knee Surg Sports Traumatol Arthrosc. 2014;22:2187–93.
73. Faul F, Erdfelder E, Lang A-G, Buchner A. G*Power: a flexible statistical power analysis program for the social, behavioral, and biomedical sciences. Behav Res Methods. 2007;39:175–91.
74. Irrgang JJ, Anderson AF, Boland AL, Harner CD, Neyret P, Richmond JC, Shelbourne KD, Bergfeld J, Feagin J, Fulkerson J, Kocher M, Howell S, Staubli H, Hefti F, Hoher J, Jacob R, Mueller W, Chan KM, Kurosaka M. Responsiveness of the international knee documentation committee subjective knee form. Am J Sports Med. 2006;34:1567–73.
75. Fanelli G, Edson C. Surgical treatment of combined PCL–ACL medial and lateral side injuries (global laxity): surgical technique and 2- to 18-year results. J Knee Surg. 2012;25:307–16.
76. Tompkins MA, Freeman AL, Hursh E, Bechtold JE. MCL internal brace does not fully recapitulate normal MCL function in valgus stress. Knee Surg Sports Traumatol Arthrosc. 2023;31(9):3604–10. https://doi.org/10.1007/s00167-023-07438-4.
77. Ateschrang A, Döbele S, Freude T, Stöckle U, Schröter S, Kraus TM. Acute MCL and ACL injuries: first results of minimal-invasive MCL ligament bracing with combined ACL single-bundle reconstruction. Arch Orthop Trauma Surg. 2016;136(9):1265–72. https://doi.org/10.1007/s00402-016-2497-6.
78. Tompkins MA, Williams H, Bechtold JE. An MCL internal brace can withstand cyclic fatigue loading and produce a valgus load to failure similar to that of intact knees. Knee Surg Sports Traumatol Arthrosc. 2023;31(9):3611–7. https://doi.org/10.1007/s00167-023-07439-3.
79. van Eck CF, Nakamura T, Price T, Linde M, Smolinski P. Suture tape augmentation improves laxity of MCL repair in the ACL reconstructed knee. Knee Surg Sports Traumatol Arthrosc. 2021;29(8):2545–52. https://doi.org/10.1007/s00167-020-06386-7.
80. Sim JA, Na YG, Choi JW, Lee BH. Early medial reconstruction combined with severely injured medial collateral ligaments can decrease residual medial laxity in anterior cruciate ligament reconstruction. Arch Orthop Trauma Surg. 2022;142(10):2791–9. https://doi.org/10.1007/s00402-021-04211-5.
81. Dong J, Ji G, Zhang Y, Gao S, Wang F, Chen B. Single allograft medial collateral ligament and posterior oblique ligament reconstruction: a technique to improve valgus and rotational stability. Eur J Orthop Surg Traumatol. 2014;24(6):1025–9. https://doi.org/10.1007/s00590-013-1265-3.
82. Van den Bogaerde JM, Shin E, Neu CP, Marder RA. The superficial medial collateral ligament reconstruction of the knee: effect of altering graft length on knee kinematics and stability. Knee Surg Sports Traumatol Arthrosc. 2011;19(Suppl 1):S60–8. https://doi.org/10.1007/s00167-011-1519-8.
83. Kittl C, Robinson J, Raschke MJ, Olbrich A, Frank A, Glasbrenner J, Herbst E, Domnick C, Herbort M. Medial collateral ligament reconstruction graft isometry is effected by femoral position more than tibial position. Knee Surg Sports Traumatol Arthrosc. 2021;29(11):3800–8. https://doi.org/10.1007/s00167-020-06420-8.
84. Lind M, Jacobsen K, Nielsen T. Medial collateral ligament (MCL) reconstruction results in improved medial stability: results from the Danish knee ligament reconstruction registry (DKRR). Knee Surg Sports Traumatol Arthrosc. 2020;28(3):881–7. https://doi.org/10.1007/s00167-019-05535-x.

85. Barrett IJ, Krych AJ, Pareek A, Johnson NR, Dahm DL, Stuart MJ, Levy BA. Short- to mid-term outcomes of anatomic MCL reconstruction with Achilles tendon allograft after multi-ligament knee injury. Knee Surg Sports Traumatol Arthrosc. 2018;26(10):2952–9. https://doi.org/10.1007/s00167-018-4843-4.

Chapter 16
Lateral Collateral Ligament Tears

Alfred J. Tria Jr. and Giles R. Scuderi

Machine Generated Summaries

Disclaimer: The summaries in this chapter were generated from Springer Nature publications using abstractive AI auto-summarization: An abstraction-based summarizer creates new text based on deep learning. New phrases are created to summarize the content. As the constituted sentences are machine selected, they may not fully reflect the body of the work, so we strongly advise that the original content is read and cited. The auto-generated summaries were curated by the editor to meet Springer Nature publication standards.

Machine generated keywords: acl, anterior, knee, footprint, tka, group, cut, graft, acl reconstruction, kinematic, tunnel, external rotation, intact knee, simulate, bone resection

Combined Anterior Cruciate and Lateral Collateral Ligaments Reconstruction with Ipsilateral Hamstring Autograft: Surgical Technique [36]

This is a machine-generated summary of:

Piedade, Sérgio Rocha; Górios, Carlos; Migliorini, Filippo; Maffulli, Nicola: Combined anterior cruciate and lateral collateral ligaments reconstruction with ipsilateral hamstring autograft: surgical technique [36]

A. J. Tria Jr. (✉)
Department of Orthopedics, Rutgers-Robert Wood Johnson Medical School, New Brunswick, NJ, USA

G. R. Scuderi
Northwell Health Orthopaedic Institute, New York, NY, USA

A. J. Tria Jr., G. R. Scuderi (eds.), *Ligaments of the Knee*,
https://doi.org/10.1007/978-3-031-66615-5_16

Published in: Journal of Orthopaedic Surgery and Research (2022)
Link to original: https://doi.org/10.1186/s13018-022-03358-0

If you want to cite the papers, please refer to the original.

For technical reasons we could not place the page where the original quote is coming from.

Research Highlights

Anterior cruciate ligament (ACL) and lateral collateral ligament (LCL) injuries are debilitating conditions that often require surgical intervention. Current reconstruction techniques, while effective, can be limited by the availability of autologous grafts, particularly in cases of multi-ligament injuries. Piedade et al. present a surgical procedure for reconstructing combined ACL and LCL injuries using ipsilateral hamstring autografts, offering a promising alternative to traditional methods.

The authors used a single femoral tunnel for both ACL and LCL reconstructions, thereby simplifying the procedure and reducing the risk of tunnel confluence. The technique involves harvesting the gracilis and semitendinosus tendons while preserving their tibial insertion, followed by preparation of bone tunnels and grafts. The authors detail the step-by-step process, from initial arthroscopic assessment to graft fixation, emphasizing the importance of adjusting tunnel diameters to match the harvested grafts. By integrating clinical assessment with advanced imaging techniques like MRI and valgus stress radiographs, the researchers ensure accurate diagnosis and tailored surgical planning.

The main advance presented in this study is the streamlined reconstruction technique that mitigates the need for multiple tendon grafts and femoral tunnels. This method not only reduces surgical complexity but also addresses limitations associated with allograft availability and donor site morbidity. As noted by the authors, this technique has become a reproducible and time-efficient procedure in their practice. Looking forward, further research could explore biomechanical outcomes associated with different graft passage directions and long-term patient recovery profiles. The authors have opened new avenues for treating complex knee ligament injuries, potentially improving access to care in resource-limited settings where allografts are scarce.

Double-Bundle Reconstruction Cannot Restore Intact Knee Kinematics in the ACL/LCL-Deficient Knee [37]

This is a machine-generated summary of:

Zantop, Thore; Schumacher, Tobias; Schanz, Steffen; Raschke, Michael J.; Petersen, Wolf: Double-bundle reconstruction cannot restore intact knee kinematics in the ACL/LCL-deficient knee [37]

Published in: Archives of Orthopaedic and Trauma Surgery (2010)

Link to original: https://doi.org/10.1007/s00402-010-1081-8

If you want to cite the papers, please refer to the original.

For technical reasons we could not place the page where the original quote is coming from.

Research Highlights

The anterior cruciate ligament (ACL) is crucial for maintaining knee stability, particularly as a primary restraint to tibial anterior translation. Despite this, ACL injuries often result in altered knee kinematics, leading to subjective instability and the "giving way" phenomenon in patients. While the pivot shift test is used clinically to assess instability, its efficacy can be compromised by additional injuries to secondary restraints or by varus malalignment. Zantop et al. address the effectiveness of single-bundle (SB) and anatomic double-bundle (DB) ACL reconstructions in restoring knee kinematics in ACL/LCL-deficient knees using a robotic/Universal force moment sensor (UFS) testing system.

The study utilized ten fresh-frozen human cadaveric knees, ensuring no prior surgical interventions or significant abnormalities. The study aimed to replicate clinical settings by simulating pivot shift tests and assessing rotational stability in vitro. The robotic/UFS testing system employed allowed for precise control and measurement of knee movements across various degrees of freedom. The researchers hypothesized that anatomic DB ACL reconstruction would more effectively restore intact knee kinematics compared to SB reconstruction, particularly in knees deficient in both ACL and lateral collateral ligament (LCL). Their surgical technique involved alternating between SB and DB reconstructions, with bone cement used to fill tunnels between procedures to prevent graft loosening. The testing protocol applied forces mimicking clinical examinations to assess anterior tibial translation (ATT) under different conditions: intact, ACL/LCL-deficient, SB ACL-reconstructed/LCL-deficient, and DB ACL-reconstructed/LCL-deficient.

Contrary to their hypothesis, Zantop found that neither SB nor DB ACL reconstructions fully restored rotational stability to the levels of an intact knee. While there was a significant difference in ATT under simulated KT tests between SB and DB reconstructions at certain flexion angles, no significant difference was observed under simulated pivot shift loads. These findings suggest that additional extra-articular injuries may influence the success of intra-articular ACL reconstructions. The extra-articular instability component seems to outrange the capacity of the intra-articular ACL reconstruction. Future research should consider strategies that address both intra- and extra-articular deficiencies for comprehensive treatment of ACL ruptures with associated lateral instability.

The Evaluation of the Distance Between the Popliteus Tendon and the Lateral Collateral Ligament Footprint and the Implant in Total Knee Arthroplasty Using a 3-Dimensional Template [38]

This is a machine-generated summary of:

Takubo, Akihito; Ryu, Keinosuke; Iriuchishima, Takanori; Nagaoka, Masahiro; Tokuhashi, Yasuaki; Aizawa, Shin: The evaluation of the distance between the popliteus tendon and the lateral collateral ligament footprint and the implant in Total knee Arthroplasty using a 3-dimensional template [38]

Published in: BMC Musculoskeletal Disorders (2020)

Link to original: https://doi.org/10.1186/s12891-020-03347-6

If you want to cite the papers, please refer to the original.

For technical reasons we could not place the page where the original quote is coming from.

Research Highlights

The popliteus tendon (PT) and the lateral collateral ligament (LCL) play crucial roles in stabilizing the knee, particularly during total knee arthroplasty (TKA), a surgical procedure with high success rates for treating osteoarthritic changes. However, the proximity of PT and LCL attachments to the femoral bone resection area during TKA poses a risk of iatrogenic injury, which has not been thoroughly evaluated in three-dimensional studies. Takubo et al. studied the distance between PT or LCL footprints and the TKA implant using a template system, aiming to inform surgical choices and minimize injury risks.

The authors utilized 18 formalin-fixed cadaveric lower limbs to conduct their research. They dissected the PT and LCL, marking their attachments with ink and K-wires for precise identification in computed tomography (CT) scans. The researchers employed Image J software for area measurements and analyzed distances using coronal and sagittal CT slices. Their approach allowed for accurate three-dimensional assessments of the relationships between ligament footprints and TKA implants. Two popular TKA models, Journey II BCS and Persona PS, were simulated within the template system to determine potential overlaps with PT and LCL footprints during surgery. The analysis included multiple measurements by different investigators to ensure reliability, followed by statistical evaluation using SPSS software.

The key advance of this study is the finding that a significant percentage of knees showed overlap between the PT footprint and TKA implants in simulations, indicating a substantial risk of iatrogenic injury during surgery. While no significant difference was found between the two implant models regarding proximity to PT or LCL footprints, these insights are critical for surgeons aiming to preserve knee stability post-TKA. This work underscores the importance of considering individual implant designs and surgical techniques to prevent damage to these vital structures. Understanding these spatial relationships can guide selection appropriate implants and planning cuts to avoid compromising knee function.Looking ahead, further research should explore long-term outcomes and knee kinematics following PT injuries due to osteotomy, as well as potential variations across different populations. Despite its limitations, such as sample size and demographic specificity, this study paves the way for more personalized and safer TKA procedures.

Relative Role Changing of Lateral Collateral Ligament on the Posterolateral Rotatory Instability According to the Knee Flexion Angles: A Biomechanical Comparative Study of Role of Lateral Collateral Ligament and Popliteofibular Ligament [39]

This is a machine-generated summary of:

Lim, Hong Chul; Bae, Ji Hoon; Bae, Tae Soo; Moon, Byung Chul; Shyam, Ashok K.; Wang, Joon Ho: Relative role changing of lateral collateral ligament on the posterolateral rotatory instability according to the knee flexion angles: a biomechanical comparative study of role of lateral collateral ligament and popliteofibular ligament [39]

Published in: Archives of Orthopaedic and Trauma Surgery (2012)

Link to original: https://doi.org/10.1007/s00402-012-1591-7

If you want to cite the papers, please refer to the original.

For technical reasons we could not place the page where the original quote is coming from.

Research Highlights

Isolated injuries to the posterolateral corner (PLC) of the knee, while rare, can lead to significant disability due to their role in stabilizing the joint against various forces. The lateral collateral ligament (LCL) and the popliteofibular ligament (PFL) are key structures in this region, with the LCL primarily resisting varus stress and the PFL and popliteus tendon (PT) limiting external tibial rotation. However, the specific contributions of these ligaments at different knee flexion angles remain unclear. Lim et al. investigate how the functional roles of the LCL and PFL change with knee flexion angles, providing insights that could influence surgical approaches to PLC injuries.

The investigators utilized eight cadaveric knee joints to simulate PLC injuries and assess ligament function. They employed a sequential sectioning technique to isolate and evaluate the LCL and PFL's individual contributions to rotational stability at varying degrees of knee flexion. By applying a consistent external rotational torque and measuring subsequent increases in tibial rotation after each ligament was cut, they quantified each structure's role. Their approach allowed for a comparative analysis between the effects of sectioning the LCL versus the PFL first, revealing nuanced insights into their relative importance across different knee positions.

The findings elucidate that both the LCL and PFL are crucial in limiting external rotation at an extended knee position, but as the knee flexes beyond 30 degrees, the PFL assumes a more dominant role. This suggests that while both ligaments are integral to knee stability, their significance varies with knee flexion angle—a fact that could have substantial implications for reconstructive surgery following PLC injuries. Future research may build on these results to refine surgical techniques further or develop new approaches that account for these dynamic changes in ligament function. As Lim et al. highlight, understanding each ligament's contribution is essential for accurately diagnosing PLC injuries and deciding whether LCL reconstruction is necessary in cases of posterolateral rotatory instability.

Isolated Distal Grade III Lateral Collateral Ligament Injury: What Is the Real Clinical Impact in Professional Athletes? [40]

This is a machine-generated summary of:

Gnesutta, Aroa; Sollami, Giulia; Calvi, Marco; Francese, Fabio; Mazzoni, Stefano; Genovese, Eugenio Annibale: Isolated distal grade III lateral collateral ligament injury: what is the real clinical impact in professional athletes? [40]

Published in: Skeletal Radiology (2023)

Link to original: https://doi.org/10.1007/s00256-023-04463-9

If you want to cite the papers, please refer to the original.

For technical reasons we could not place the page where the original quote is coming from.

Research Highlights

The lateral collateral ligament (LCL) is a critical component in maintaining the stability of the knee, particularly against varus forces and external rotation. Despite its importance, isolated injuries to the LCL are uncommon and often overshadowed by concurrent damage to other knee structures, leading to challenges in diagnosis and management. Gnesutta et al. present cases of professional soccer players with isolated distal LCL grade III injuries who were successfully managed conservatively, challenging the traditional surgical approach.

The investigators focused on three professional soccer players who sustained direct varus force trauma during matches. Utilizing a 1.5-Tesla MRI system with a dedicated knee coil, the team conducted a thorough imaging protocol that included sagittal TSE and SPAIR sequences; coronal SPAIR sequence; and axial TSE sequence. The MRIs were evaluated by an experienced radiologist, revealing isolated LCL III grade injuries characterized by complete ligament tears with significant surrounding edema. Remarkably, these athletes returned to competitive play without surgery, relying solely on clinical follow-up and targeted physical therapy.

The study's narrative is built upon the detailed imaging features that contributed to accurate diagnoses and the conservative management strategies employed. Gnesutta emphasizes the potential for non-surgical treatment in certain cases of severe LCL injury, which could have significant implications for sports medicine and orthopedic practice.

The successful return of professional athletes to high-level competition following conservative treatment of grade III LCL injuries suggests that non-operative approaches may be more viable than previously thought. The results invites reconsideration of the LCL's role in knee stabilization. This study not only contributes valuable clinical insights but also highlights the need for further research involving larger patient cohorts and direct comparisons between surgical and non-surgical outcomes to optimize treatment strategies for isolated LCL injuries.

Bibliography

1. Dean RS, LaPrade RF. ACL and posterolateral corner injuries. Curr Rev Musculoskelet Med. 2020;13(1):123–32. https://doi.org/10.1007/s12178-019-09581-3.
2. Stevens KJ, Dragoo JL. Anterior cruciate ligament tears and associated injuries. Top Magn Reson Imaging. 2006;17(5):347–62. https://doi.org/10.1097/RMR.0b013e3180421cc2.
3. Dekker TJ, Schairer WW, Grantham WJ, DePhillipo NN, Aman ZS, LaPrade RF. Fibular collateral ligament reconstruction graft options: clinical and radiographic outcomes of autograft versus allograft. Arthroscopy. 2021;37(3):944–50. https://doi.org/10.1016/j.arthro.2020.10.034.
4. Niki Y, Matsumoto H, Otani T, et al. A modified Larson's method of posterolateral corner reconstruction of the knee reproducing the physiological tensioning pattern of the lateral collateral and popliteofibular ligaments. BMC Sports Sci Med Rehabil. 2012;4:21. https://doi.org/10.1186/1758-2555-4-21.
5. LaPrade RF, Spiridonov SI, Coobs BR, Ruckert PR, Griffith CJ. Fibular collateral ligament anatomical reconstructions: a prospective outcomes study. Am J Sports Med. 2010;38(10):2005–11. https://doi.org/10.1177/0363546510370200.
6. Noyes FR, Barber-Westin SD. Reconstruction of the lateral collateral ligament of the knee with patellar tendon allograft. Report of a new technique in combined ligament injuries. Am J Sports Med. 1999;27(2):269–70.
7. Liu P, Wang J, Zhao F, Xu Y, Ao Y. Anatomic, arthroscopically assisted, mini-open fibular collateral ligament reconstruction: an in vitro biomechanical study. Am J Sports Med. 2014;42(2):373–81. https://doi.org/10.1177/0363546513508536.
8. Kennedy MI, Bernhardson A, Moatshe G, Buckley PS, Engebretsen L, LaPrade RF. Fibular collateral ligament/posterolateral corner injury: when to repair, reconstruct, or both. Clin Sports Med. 2019;38(2):261–74. https://doi.org/10.1016/j.csm.2018.11.002.
9. Fanelli GC. Surgical reconstruction for acute posterolateral injury of the knee. J Knee Surg. 2005;18:157–62.
10. Kim YC, Chung IH, Yoo WK, Shu JS, Kim SJ, Park CI. Anatomic and magnetic resonance imaging of the posterolateral structures of the knee. Clin Anat. 1997;10:397–404.
11. Lipke JM, Janecki CJ, Nelson CL, McLeod P, Thompson C, Thompson J, Haynes DW. The role of incompetence of the anterior cruciate and lateral ligaments in anterolateral and anteromedial instability. A biomechanical study of cadaver knees. J Bone Jt Surg Am. 1981;63:954–60.
12. Markolf KL, Mensch JS, Amstutz HC. Stiffness and laxity of the knee—the contributions of the supporting structures. A quantitative in vitro study. J Bone Jt Surg Am. 1976;58A:583–94.
13. Seering WP, Piziali RL, Nagel DA, Schurman DJ. The function of the primary ligaments of the knee in varus–valgus and axial rotation. J Biomech. 1980;13:785–94.
14. Covey DC. Current concepts review: injuries of the posterolateral corner of the knee. J Bone Jt Surg. 2001;83:106–18.
15. Staubli HU, Birrer S. The popliteus tendon and its fascicles at the popliteal hiatus: gross anatomy and functional arthroscopic evaluation with and without anterior cruciate ligament deficiency. Arthroscopy. 1990;6:209–20.

16. Vogrin TM, Hoher J, Aroen A, Woo SL, Harner CD. Effects of sectioning the posterolateral structures on knee kinematics and in situ forces in the posterior cruciate ligament. Knee Surg Sports Traumatol Arthrosc. 2000;8:93–8.
17. Zantop T, Schumacher T, Diermann N, Schanz S, Raschke MJ, Petersen W. Anterolateral rotational knee instability: role of posterolateral structures. Arch Orthop Trauma Surg. 2007;127(9):743–52.
18. Slocum DB, Larson RL. Rotatory instability of the knee. Its pathogenesis and a clinical test to demonstrate its presence. J Bone Jt Surg. 1968;50:211–25.
19. Zantop T, Mirko H, Weimann Andre F, Freddie H, Wolf P. The role of anteromedial and posterolateral bundle of the ACL in anterior tibial translation and internal rotation. Am J Sports Med. 2007;35(2):223–7.
20. Zantop T, Petersen W, Sekiya JK, Musahl V, Fu FH. Anterior cruciate ligament anatomy and function relating to anatomical reconstruction. Knee Surg Sports Traumatol Arthrosc. 2006;14(10):982–92.
21. Cha PS, Brucker PU, West RV, Fu FH. Arthroscopic double bundle anterior cruciate ligament reconstruction: an anatomic approach. Arthroscopy. 2005;21:1275–81.
22. Petersen W, Tretow H, Weimann A, Herbort M, Fu FH, Raschke MJ, Zantop T. Biomechanical evaluation of two techniques for double bundle ACL reconstruction using a robotic/UFS testing system. Am J Sports Med. 2007;35(2):228–34.
23. Yagi M, Wong EK, Kanamori A, Debski RE, Fu FH, Woo SL. Biomechanical analysis of an anatomic anterior cruciate ligament reconstruction. Am J Sports Med. 2002;30:660–6.
24. Yasuda K, Kondo E, Ichiyama H, Tanabe Y, Tohyama H. Clinical evaluation of anatomic double-bundle anterior cruciate ligament reconstruction procedure using hamstring tendon grafts: comparisons among 3 different procedures. Arthroscopy. 2006;22(3):240–51.
25. Aki T, Sugita T, Takahashi A, Aizawa T, Kamimura M, Sasaki A, Miyatake N, Itoi E. Femoral footprint of the popliteus tendon may be at the risk of damage during total knee arthroplasty. Knee Surg Sports Traumatol Arthrosc. 2017;25(12):3718–22.
26. Takahashi A, Sugita T, Aizawa T, Chiba D, Kamimura M, Aki T, Itoi E. Potential risk of excising the femoral insertion of the popliteus tendon during primary total knee arthroplasty: a biometric study. J Orthop Sci. 2015;20(6):1030–5.
27. Chun YM, Kim SJ, Kim HS. Evaluation of the mechanical properties of posterolateral structures and supporting posterolateral instability of the knee. J Orthop Res. 2008;26:1371–6.
28. Ricchetti ET, Sennett BJ, Huffman GR. Acute and chronic management of posterolateral corner injuries of the knee. Orthopedics. 2008;31:479–88. quiz 489–490.
29. Sugita T, Amis AA. Anatomic and biomechanical study of the lateral collateral and popliteofibular ligaments. Am J Sports Med. 2001;29:466–72.
30. Pasque C, Noyes FR, Gibbons M, Levy M, Grood E. The role of the popliteofibular ligament and the tendon of popliteus in providing stability in the human knee. J Bone Joint Surg Br. 2003;85-B:292–8.
31. Gollehon DL, Torzilli PA, Warren RF. The role of the posterolateral and cruciate ligaments in the stability of the human knee: a biomechanical study. J Bone Joint Surg Am. 1987;69:233–42.
32. Veltri DM, Deng XH, Torzilli PA, Warren RF, Maynard MJ. The role of the cruciate and posterolateral ligaments in stability of the knee: a biomechanical study. Am J Sports Med. 1995;23:436–43.
33. Grawe B, Schroeder AJ, Kakazu R, Messer MS. Lateral collateral ligament injury about the knee: anatomy, evaluation, and management. J Am Acad Orthop Surg. 2018;26(6):e120–7. https://doi.org/10.5435/JAAOS-D-16-00028.
34. Bushnell BD, Bitting SS, Crain JM, Boublik M, Schlegel TF. Treatment of magnetic resonance imaging-documented isolated grade III lateral collateral ligament injuries in National Football League athletes. Am J Sports Med. 2010;38(1):86–91. https://doi.org/10.1177/0363546509344075.

35. Davenport D, Arora A, Edwards MR. Non-operative management of an isolated lateral collateral ligament injury in an adolescent patient and review of the literature. BMJ Case Rep. 2018;2017:223478. https://doi.org/10.1136/bcr-2017-223478.
36. Piedade SR, Górios C, Migliorini F, Maffulli N. Combined anterior cruciate and lateral collateral ligaments reconstruction with ipsilateral hamstring autograft: surgical technique. J Orthop Surg Res. 2022;17:466. https://doi.org/10.1186/s13018-022-03358-0.
37. Zantop T, Schumacher T, Schanz S, Raschke MJ, Petersen W. Double-bundle reconstruction cannot restore intact knee kinematics in the ACL/LCL-deficient knee. Arch Orthop Trauma Surg. 2010;130:1019–26. https://doi.org/10.1007/s00402-010-1081-8.
38. Takubo A, Ryu K, Iriuchishima T, Nagaoka M, Tokuhashi Y, Aizawa S. The evaluation of the distance between the popliteus tendon and the lateral collateral ligament footprint and the implant in Total knee Arthroplasty using a 3-dimensional template. BMC Musculoskelet Disord. 2020;21:322. https://doi.org/10.1186/s12891-020-03347-6.
39. Lim HC, Bae JH, Bae TS, Moon BC, Shyam AK, Wang JH. Relative role changing of lateral collateral ligament on the posterolateral rotatory instability according to the knee flexion angles: a biomechanical comparative study of role of lateral collateral ligament and popliteofibular ligament. Arch Orthop Trauma Surg. 2012;132:1631–6. https://doi.org/10.1007/s00402-012-1591-7.
40. Gnesutta A, Sollami G, Calvi M, Francese F, Mazzoni S, Genovese EA. Isolated distal grade III lateral collateral ligament injury: what is the real clinical impact in professional athletes? Skeletal Radiol. 2023;53:983–7. https://doi.org/10.1007/s00256-023-04463-9.

Chapter 17
Complex Ligament Tears

Alfred J. Tria Jr. and Giles R. Scuderi

Machine Generated Summaries

Disclaimer: The summaries in this chapter were generated from Springer Nature publications using abstractive AI auto-summarization: An abstraction-based summarizer creates new text based on deep learning. New phrases are created to summarize the content. As the constituted sentences are machine selected, they may not fully reflect the body of the work, so we strongly advise that the original content is read and cited. The auto-generated summaries were curated by the editor to meet Springer Nature publication standards.

Machine generated keywords: brace, internal, internal brace, ligament brace, dislocation, mcl, knee dislocation, valgus, group, tear, acute, combine, multiligament, mlki, multiple ligament

Results of Multiple Ligament Reconstruction After Knee Dislocation——A Prospective Study with 95 Patients and Minimum 2-Year Follow Up [57]

This is a machine-generated summary of:

Li, Tao; Xiong, Yan; Zhang, Zhong; Tang, Xin; Chen, Gang; Li, Qi; Fu, Wei Li; Li, Jian: Results of multiple ligament reconstruction after knee dislocation——A prospective study with 95 patients and minimum 2-year follow up [57]

A. J. Tria Jr. (✉)
Department of Orthopedics, Rutgers-Robert Wood Johnson Medical School, New Brunswick, NJ, USA

G. R. Scuderi
Northwell Health Orthopaedic Institute, New York, NY, USA

A. J. Tria Jr., G. R. Scuderi (eds.), *Ligaments of the Knee*,
https://doi.org/10.1007/978-3-031-66615-5_17

Published in: BMC Musculoskeletal Disorders (2021)
Link to original: https://doi.org/10.1186/s12891-021-04596-9

If you want to cite the papers, please refer to the original.

For technical reasons we could not place the page where the original quote is coming from.

Research Highlights

Multiple ligament injuries represent a formidable challenge in sports medicine, with a prevalence of 0.02–0.2% of orthopedic injuries and <0.5% of all joint dislocations. Vascular injury occurs in 7–32% of these cases, while associated injuries such as common fibular nerve damage, fractures, and meniscus tears complicate the clinical picture. Li et al. developed a comprehensive classification system for multiple ligament injuries that takes into account the stage of injury and associated complications, leading to tailored treatment protocols that have shown significant functional improvements in patients.

The authors conducted a prospective study enrolling patients with multiple ligament injuries treated according to the stage-specific protocols they developed. The classification system introduced by the investigators considers not only the timing of the injury (emergency, acute, subacute, and chronic stages) but also the nature and location of ligament damage and associated fractures or other complications. This approach allowed for more individualized management strategies, which were crucial given the variability in injury patterns among patients. All participants underwent preoperative examinations using X-ray and MRI, as well as angiography when vascular damage was suspected. Surgical techniques were adapted to each case's specifics, with particular attention paid to the order of ligament reconstruction—a critical factor in treatment efficacy. Postoperative rehabilitation protocols emphasized gradual weight-bearing and range of motion exercises tailored to each patient's recovery stage.

The key advance from this research lies in its holistic approach to classifying and treating multiple ligament injuries. By integrating factors such as injury stage, associated complications, and specific ligament damage into their classification system, the authors have provided a more effective framework for managing these complex cases. This new classification can better identify the severity of the injury to plan appropriate management. The study suggests that patients treated acutely exhibit better outcomes than those in chronic stages, underscoring the importance of timely intervention. While further research with larger cohorts is necessary to validate these results fully, this study represents a significant step forward in optimizing treatment for multiple ligament injuries.

Outcomes of Multiligament Knee Injury Treated with Versus Without Internal Brace Suture Augmentation [58]

This is a machine-generated summary of:

Korber, Shane S.; Fathi, Amir; Bolia, Ioanna K.; Panish, Brian J.; Benvegnu, Neilen; Juhan, Tristan W.; Weber, Alexander E.; Argintar, Evan H.; Hatch, George F.: Outcomes of multiligament knee injury treated with versus without internal brace suture augmentation [58]

Published in: European Journal of Orthopaedic Surgery & Traumatology (2023)

Link to original: https://doi.org/10.1007/s00590-023-03575-1

If you want to cite the papers, please refer to the original.

For technical reasons we could not place the page where the original quote is coming from.

Research Highlights

Multiligament knee injuries (MLKI) present a complex challenge in orthopedic surgery, with treatment strategies evolving to improve patient outcomes. The use of internal bracing—a technique involving sutures to augment ligament repairs—has shown promise in individual ligament injuries, yet comparative studies for MLKI are scarce. Korber et al. compare the outcomes and reoperation rates of MLKI patients treated with and without internal brace augmentation.

The investigators conducted a retrospective chart review of patients who underwent surgical management for MLKI at two institutions, focusing on those treated with internal bracing from its introduction in 2016 to the present. The study included patients over 18 years old with at least 1 year of follow-up, excluding those with previous knee surgeries or nonoperative treatment for MLKI. Outcomes were assessed using validated instruments like the Lysholm Knee score and the Multiligament Quality of Life questionnaire. Surgical techniques were consistent across both internal brace and non-internal brace groups, ensuring comparability. Statistical analysis revealed no significant differences in patient-reported outcomes or reoperation rates between the two groups, although the study was underpowered.

The findings suggest that internal bracing may be as effective as traditional methods for treating MLKI, without increasing the risk of reoperation. Despite the limitations of an underpowered study and the inherent variability in MLKI cases, these findings contribute insights into surgical options for these complex injuries. The trend towards non-inferiority supports the potential utility of internal bracing, indicating a direction for future research to establish more definitive evidence through larger, matched cohort studies that could further elucidate the clinical benefits of this technique in managing MLKI.

Two-Stage Ligament Reconstruction with Remnant Preservation as Treatment of Knee Dislocation [59]

This is a machine-generated summary of:

Ma, Wenpu; Yang, Yiqun; Ha, Xin: Two-stage ligament reconstruction with remnant preservation as treatment of knee dislocation [59]

Published in: BMC Surgery (2023)

Link to original: https://doi.org/10.1186/s12893-023-02271-5

If you want to cite the papers, please refer to the original.

For technical reasons we could not place the page where the original quote is coming from.

Research Highlights

Knee dislocations are severe injuries often resulting from high-energy trauma, such as car accidents or sports collisions. These dislocations can lead to complex vascular, neurological, and multi-ligamentous damage, necessitating prompt and precise clinical management to prevent limb loss. Despite advancements in arthroscopic surgery for cruciate ligament reconstruction, there remains a lack of consensus on the optimal treatment approach, with some patients still facing long-term functional limitations. Ma et al. explore the efficacy of a two-stage reconstruction strategy with remnant preservation for treating knee dislocation, potentially offering improved outcomes for patients.

The investigators conducted a randomized controlled trial comparing two groups: one undergoing remnant-preserved reconstruction and another receiving standard reconstruction without remnant preservation. The study subjects divided patients into two groups based on the surgical technique applied. The first phase involved collateral ligament repair, followed by a waiting period to allow for recovery of knee flexion and extension before proceeding to the second phase—arthroscopic reconstruction of the anterior and posterior cruciate ligaments (ACL/PCL). The authors described their surgical methods, emphasizing the preservation of ligament remnants to enhance graft revascularization and biomechanical properties. They also detailed postoperative rehabilitation protocols designed to protect the reconstructed ligaments and promote healing.

The study demonstrated that two-stage reconstruction with remnant preservation significantly improves postoperative knee function compared to traditional methods. Patients in the remnant-preserved group showed better knee flexion angles and higher scores on various functional assessments at follow-up. These findings suggest that preserving ligament remnants during ACL/PCL reconstruction could be crucial for restoring joint stability and improving clinical outcomes after knee dislocation.

Anatomic Repair and Ligament Bracing as an Alternative Treatment Option for Acute Combined PCL Injuries Involving the Posteromedial or Posterolateral Corner—Results of a Multicentre Study [60]

This is a machine-generated summary of:

Gensior, Tobias J.; Mester, Bastian; Achtnich, Andrea; Winkler, Philipp W.; Henkelmann, Ralf; Hepp, Pierre; Glaab, Richard; Krause, Matthias; Frosch, Karl-Heinz; Zellner, Johannes; Schoepp, Christian: Anatomic repair and ligament bracing as an alternative treatment option for acute combined PCL injuries involving the posteromedial or posterolateral corner—results of a multicentre study [60]

Published in: Archives of Orthopaedic and Trauma Surgery (2023)
Link to original: https://doi.org/10.1007/s00402-023-05015-5

If you want to cite the papers, please refer to the original.

For technical reasons we could not place the page where the original quote is coming from.

Research Highlights

The management of posterior cruciate ligament (PCL) injuries, particularly when combined with collateral ligament complexes, remains a subject of debate in orthopedic surgery. While non-operative treatment is favored for isolated PCL tears due to their intrinsic healing potential, the presence of additional ligamentous injuries often necessitates surgical intervention. However, the optimal surgical technique for acute combined PCL injuries involving the posteromedial (PMC) or posterolateral corner (PLC) of the knee is not well-defined, with limited evidence guiding the decision between primary suture repair with or without ligament bracing and primary ligament reconstruction. Gensior et al. evaluate the clinical outcomes of a single-stage augmented primary suture repair technique in patients with acute combined PCL injuries.

The investigators conducted a multicenter study across six trauma centers in Germany, where patients with acute combined PCL injuries underwent one-stage suture repair with additional suture augmentation by ligament bracing. The study included patients who were operated on within 14 days of injury and excluded those with additional ACL injuries or knee dislocations. The authors hypothesized that this approach would yield favorable clinical and radiological outcomes similar to those observed in knee dislocation treatments. The surgical strategy involved arthroscopic PCL bracing and repair/refixation of injured peripheral structures, followed by an individualized rehabilitation protocol based on the presence of intraarticular pathologies.

The study included 31 patients with combined PCL injuries (female: male = 7:24; age 39.1 ± 13.8 years) with a follow-up of 16.8 ± 9.6 months were finally evaluated. 18 had PMC injuries, 13 PLC injuries. 32.2% presented with accompanying meniscal tears (70% medial meniscus). 19.4% showed cartilage injuries grade III-IV. Complications included one infection and four knee stiffnesses. Three had symptomatic postoperative instability, all affiliated to the PLC group. The IKDC was 69.8 ± 16.5, Lysholm score 85 ± 14.4 and KOOS 89.7 ± 8.1. Median loss of activity (Tegner) was 0.89 ± 1.31. Comparing PMC and PLC, all scores showed a tendency towards more favorable outcomes in the PMC group (n.s.). Stress-radiography showed an overall side-to-side difference of 3.7 ± 3.8 mm. Subgroup evaluation showed statistically significant better results (p = 0.035) of PMC (2.5 ± 1.5 mm) versus PLC (5.8 ± 5.6 mm).

This study represents a significant advance in the treatment of acute combined PCL injuries, demonstrating that one-stage suture repair with ligament bracing can lead to good to excellent clinical outcomes. Patients with PMC injuries tended to have more reliable results compared to those with PLC injuries. This research suggests that this surgical technique is a viable option for managing such complex knee injuries. Future research could focus on larger patient populations to confirm these findings and further compare outcomes between different surgical techniques within the PLC group.

Acute MCL and ACL Injuries: First Results of Minimal-Invasive MCL Ligament Bracing with Combined ACL Single-Bundle Reconstruction [61]

This is a machine-generated summary of:

Ateschrang, A.; Döbele, S.; Freude, T.; Stöckle, U.; Schröter, S.; Kraus, T. M.: Acute MCL and ACL injuries: first results of minimal-invasive MCL ligament bracing with combined ACL single-bundle reconstruction [61]

Published in: Archives of Orthopaedic and Trauma Surgery (2016)

Link to original: https://doi.org/10.1007/s00402-016-2497-6

If you want to cite the papers, please refer to the original.

For technical reasons we could not place the page where the original quote is coming from.

Research Highlights

Injuries to the medial collateral ligament (MCL) frequently accompany anterior cruciate ligament (ACL) tears, presenting a complex challenge in orthopedic sports medicine. While the MCL has shown good healing potential, its treatment in conjunction with ACL injuries remains debated, with concerns that improper stability may compromise ACL reconstruction. Ateschrang et al. introduces a minimal-invasive technique for MCL bracing combined with ACL reconstruction, aiming to improve postoperative stability and reduce complications such as joint stiffness from arthrofibrosis.

The study involved patients who underwent surgery within days of injury, using a minimal-invasive ligament bracing technique for the MCL and a single-bundle technique for the ACL reconstruction. The authors detailed their methods, from patient selection criteria—acute complete rupture of the ACL with grade II° or III° valgus laxity—to the surgical procedure itself. The MCL stabilization involved securing the ligament with an ultrahigh-molecular-weight polyethylene tape, anchored without extensive soft tissue damage, thus preserving knee structures and potentially reducing recovery complications. Postoperative care followed standardized protocols, and outcomes were measured through various clinical assessments including Lachman test, Rolimeter™ for sagittal stability, and subjective scoring systems like Lysholm and Tegner scores.

The study demonstrated that acute combined ACL and MCL lesions can be effectively managed through this surgical technique, yielding biomechanically stable knees with promising clinical outcomes. Notably, the incidence of postoperative arthrofibrosis was low at 0%, suggesting that this approach may mitigate one of the primary concerns associated with combined ligament surgeries. These findings contribute valuable insights into the treatment of complex knee injuries, though they acknowledge limitations such as small sample size and lack of a control group.

Bibliography

1. Howells NR, Brunton LR, Robinson J, Porteus AJ, Eldridge JD, Murray JR. Acute knee dislocation: an evidence based approach to the management of the multiligament injured knee. Injury. 2011;42(11):1198–204. https://doi.org/10.1016/j.injury.2010.11.018.
2. Natsuhara KM, Yeranosian MG, Cohen JR, Wang JC, McAllister DR, Petrigliano FA. What is the frequency of vascular injury after knee dislocation? Clin Orthop Relat Res. 2014;472(9):2615–20. https://doi.org/10.1007/s11999-014-3566-1.
3. Liu X, Feng H, Zhang H, Hong L, Wang XS, Zhang J, et al. Surgical treatment of subacute and chronic valgus instability in multiligament-injured knees with superficial medial collateral ligament reconstruction using Achilles allografts: a quantitative analysis with a minimum 2-year follow-up. Am J Sports Med. 2013;41(5):1044–50. https://doi.org/10.1177/0363546513479016.
4. Rihn JA, Groff YJ, Harner CD, Cha PS. The acutely dislocated knee: evaluation and management. J Am Acad Orthop Surg. 2004;12(5):334–46. https://doi.org/10.5435/00124635-200409000-00008.
5. Robertson A, Nutton RW, Keating JF. Dislocation of the knee. J Bone Joint Surg (Br). 2006;88(6):706–11.
6. Hirschmann MT, Hoffmann M, Krause R, Jenabzadeh RA, Arnold MP, Friederich NF. Anterolateral approach with tibial tubercle osteotomy versus standard medial approach for primary total knee arthroplasty: does it matter? BMC Musculoskelet Disord. 2010;11(1):167. https://doi.org/10.1186/1471-2474-11-167.
7. Hirschmann MT, Iranpour F, Muller W, Friederich NF. Surgical treatment of complex bicruciate knee ligament injuries in elite athletes: what long-term outcome can we expect? Am J Sports Med. 2010;38(6):1103–9. https://doi.org/10.1177/0363546509356978.
8. Hirschmann MT, Zimmermann N, Rychen T, Candrian C, Hudetz D, Lorez LG, et al. Clinical and radiological outcomes after management of traumatic knee dislocation by open single

stage complete reconstruction/repair. BMC Musculoskelet Disord. 2010;11(1):102. https://doi.org/10.1186/1471-2474-11-102.

9. Levy BA, Dajani KA, Whelan DB, Stannard JP, Fanelli GC, Stuart MJ, et al. Decision making in the multiligament-injured knee: an evidence-based systematic review. Arthroscopy. 2009;25(4):430–8. https://doi.org/10.1016/j.arthro.2009.01.008.
10. Darabos N, Gusic N, Vlahovic T, Darabos A, Popovic I, Vlahovic I. Staged management of knee dislocation in polytrauma injured patients. Injury. 2013;44(Suppl 3):S40–5. https://doi.org/10.1016/S0020-1383(13)70196-7.
11. Bonnevialle P, Chaufour X, Loustau O, Mansat P, Pidhorz L, Mansat M. Traumatic knee dislocation with popliteal vascular disruption: retrospective study of 14 cases. Rev Chir Orthop Reparatrice Appar Mot. 2006;92(8):768–77. https://doi.org/10.1016/S0035-1040(06)75945-1.
12. Kohl S, Stock A, Ahmad SS, Zumstein M, Keel M, Exadaktylos A, et al. Dynamic intraligamentary stabilization and primary repair: a new concept for the treatment of knee dislocation. Injury. 2015;46(4):724–8. https://doi.org/10.1016/j.injury.2014.10.012.
13. Moatshe G, Dornan GJ, Ludvigsen T, Loken S, LaPrade RF, Engebretsen L. High prevalence of knee osteoarthritis at a minimum 10-year follow-up after knee dislocation surgery. Knee Surg Sports Traumatol Arthrosc. 2017;25(12):3914–22. https://doi.org/10.1007/s00167-017-4443-8.
14. Ranger P, Senay A, Gratton GR, Lacelle M, Delisle J. LARS synthetic ligaments for the acute management of 111 acute knee dislocations: effective surgical treatment for most ligaments. Knee Surg Sports Traumatol Arthrosc. 2018;26(12):3673–81. https://doi.org/10.1007/s00167-018-4940-4.
15. Fanelli GC, Sousa PL, Edson CJ. Long-term followup of surgically treated knee dislocations: stability restored, but arthritis is common. Clin Orthop Relat Res. 2014;472(9):2712–7. https://doi.org/10.1007/s11999-014-3707-6.
16. Engebretsen L, Risberg MA, Robertson B, Ludvigsen TC, Johansen S. Outcome after knee dislocations: a 2-9 years follow-up of 85 consecutive patients. Knee Surg Sports Traumatol Arthrosc. 2009;17(9):1013–26. https://doi.org/10.1007/s00167-009-0869-y.
17. Angelini FJ, Helito CP, Bonadio MB, da Mota EARF, Pecora JR, Camanho GL. Surgical management of knee dislocations with ligament reconstruction associated with a hinged external fixator. Orthop Traumatol Surg Res. 2015;101(1):77–81. https://doi.org/10.1016/j.otsr.2014.11.001.
18. Stannard JP, Nuelle CW, McGwin G, Volgas DA. Hinged external fixation in the treatment of knee dislocations: a prospective randomized study. J Bone Joint Surg Am. 2014;96(3):184–91. https://doi.org/10.2106/JBJS.L.01603.
19. Wilson WT, Hopper GP, Byrne PA, MacKay GM. Anterior cruciate ligament repair with internal brace ligament augmentation. Surg Technol Int. 2016;29:273–8.
20. McIntyre V, Hopper GP, Mackay GM. Anterior cruciate ligament repair in a professional soccer player using internal brace ligament augmentation: a case report focusing on rehabilitation. Surg Technol Int. 2019;35:341–8.
21. Rothfeld A, Pawlak A, Liebler SAH, Morris M, Paci JM. Patellar tendon repair augmentation with a knotless suture anchor internal brace: a biomechanical cadaveric study. Am J Sports Med. 2018;46(5):1199–204. https://doi.org/10.1177/0363546517751916.
22. Ko PY, Huang MT, Li CL, Su WR, Jou IM, Wu PT. Jigless knotless internal brace technique for acute achilles tendon rupture: a case series study. J Orthop Surg Res. 2019;14(1):415. https://doi.org/10.1186/s13018-019-1471-8.
23. Heitmann M, Akoto R, Krause M, Hepp P, Schopp C, Gensior TJ, et al. Management of acute knee dislocations: anatomic repair and ligament bracing as a new treatment option-results of a multicentre study. Knee Surg Sports Traumatol Arthrosc. 2019;27(8):2710–8. https://doi.org/10.1007/s00167-018-5317-4.
24. Hanley JM, Anthony CA, DeMik D, Glass N, Amendola A, Wolf BR, Bollier M. Patient-reported outcomes after multiligament knee injury: mcl repair versus reconstruction. Orthop J Sports Med. 2017;5(3):2325967117694818. https://doi.org/10.1177/2325967117694818.

25. Jonkergouw A, van der List JP, DiFelice GS. Multiligament repair with suture augmentation in a knee dislocation with medial-sided injury. Arthrosc Tech. 2018;7(8):e839–43. https://doi.org/10.1016/j.eats.2018.04.006.
26. Lee JH-Y, Cook JL, Wilson N, Rucinski K, Stannard JP. Outcomes after multiligament knee injury reconstruction using novel graft constructs and techniques. J Knee Surg. 2020;35(05):502–10. https://doi.org/10.1055/s-0040-1716356.
27. Trasolini NA, Korber S, Gipsman A, San AE, Weber AE, Hatch GFR III. Performance of PROMIS computer adaptive testing as compared with established instruments for multiple-ligament knee injuries. Orthop J Sports Med. 2019;7(9):2325967119867419.
28. Arciero RA. Anatomic posterolateral corner knee reconstruction. Arthroscopy. 2005;21(9):1147. https://doi.org/10.1016/j.arthro.2005.06.008.
29. LaPrade RF, Johansen S, Wentorf FA, Engebretsen L, Esterberg JL, Tso A. An analysis of an anatomical posterolateral knee reconstruction: an in vitro biomechanical study and development of a surgical technique. Am J Sports Med. 2004;32(6):1405–14. https://doi.org/10.1177/0363546503262687.
30. Borden PS, Kantaras AT, Caborn DN. Medial collateral ligament reconstruction with allograft using a double-bundle technique. Arthroscopy. 2002;18(4):E19. https://doi.org/10.1053/jars.2002.32235.
31. Dong JT, Chen BC, Men XQ, Wang F, Hao JD, Zhao JN, Wang XF, Zhang XY, Sun R. Application of triangular vector to functionally reconstruct the medial collateral ligament with double bundle allograft technique. Arthrosc J Arthrosc Relat Surg. 2012;28(10):1445–53.
32. Lind M, Jakobsen BW, Lund B, Hansen MS, Abdallah O, Christiansen SE. Anatomical reconstruction of the medial collateral ligament and posteromedial corner of the knee in patients with chronic medial collateral ligament instability. Am J Sports Med. 2009;37(6):1116–22. https://doi.org/10.1177/0363546509332498.
33. Gilmer BB, Crall T, DeLong J, Kubo T, Mackay G, Jani SS. Biomechanical analysis of internal bracing for treatment of medial knee injuries. Orthopedics. 2016;39(3):e532–7. https://doi.org/10.3928/01477447-20160427-13.
34. Otto A, Helal A, Imhoff FB, Mehl J, Herbst E, Achtnich AE, Forkel P, Imhoff AB, Schmitt A. Promising clinical and magnetic resonance imaging results after internal bracing of acute posterior cruciate ligament lesions in multiple injured knees. Knee Surg Sports Traumatol Arthrosc. 2020;28(8):2543–50. https://doi.org/10.1007/s00167-020-05852-6.
35. Li C, Liu Y, Zheng R, Sun J, Peng W, Deng XH, et al. One-stage arthroscopic multiple ligament reconstruction for Schenck IV knee dislocation. Orthop Surg. 2023;15(2):502–9.
36. Hua W, Liu S, Wang B. Short-term effectiveness of one-stage anterior and posterior cruciate ligaments and posterolateral complex reconstruction combined with medial collateral ligament repair for KD-IV knee dislocation. Zhongguo Xiu Fu Chong Jian Wai Ke Za Zhi. 2022;36(1):10–7.
37. Ohkoshi Y, Nagasaki S, Shibata N, Yamamoto K, Hashimoto T, Yamane S. Two-stage reconstruction with autografts for knee dislocations. Clin Orthop Relat Res. 2002;398:169–75.
38. Khan MJ, Asif N, Sharma A, Siddiqui YS, Khan AQ. Single-stage versus two-stage reconstruction in chronic multi ligament knee injury. Int J Burns Trauma. 2022;12(2):35–44.
39. Adachi N, Ochi M, Uchio Y, Sumen Y. Anterior cruciate ligament augmentation under arthroscopy. A minimum 2-year follow-up in 40 patients. Arch Orthop Trauma Surg. 2000;120(3–4):128–33.
40. Lee BI, Kwon SW, Kim JB, Choi HS, Min KD. Comparison of clinical results according to amount of preserved remnant in arthroscopic anterior cruciate ligament reconstruction using quadrupled hamstring graft. Arthroscopy. 2008;24(5):560–8.
41. Jung YB, Jung HJ, Siti HT, Lee YS, Lee HJ, Lee SH, et al. Comparison of anterior cruciate ligament reconstruction with preservation only versus remnant tensioning technique. Arthroscopy. 2011;27(9):1252–8.

42. Chahla J, Murray IR, Robinson J, et al. Posterolateral corner of the knee: an expert consensus statement on diagnosis, classification, treatment, and rehabilitation. Knee Surg Sports Traumatol Arthrosc. 2019;27:2520–9. https://doi.org/10.1007/s00167-018-5260-4.
43. Frosch KPA, Heider S, Stengel D, Wohlmuth P, Hoffmann M, et al. Primary ligament sutures as a treatment option of knee dislocations: a meta-analysis. Knee Surg Sports Traumatol Arthrosc. 2013;21(7):1502–9. https://doi.org/10.1007/s00167-012-2154-8.
44. Heitmann M, Gerau M, Hötzel J, et al. Ligament bracing—Augmentierte Primärnaht bei multiligamentären Verletzungen des Kniegelenks. Oper Orthop Traumatol. 2014;26:19–29. https://doi.org/10.1007/s00064-013-0263-2.
45. Duncan JB, Hunter R, Purnell M, Freeman J. Meniscal injuries associated with acute anterior cruciate ligament tears in alpine skiers. Am J Sports Med. 1995;23(2):170–2.
46. Zaffagnini S, Bignozzi S, Martelli S, Lopomo N, Marcacci M. Does ACL reconstruction restore knee stability in combined lesions?: an in vivo study. Clin Orthop Relat Res. 2007;454:95–9.
47. Abramowitch SD, Yagi M, Tsuda E, Woo SL. The healing medial collateral ligament following a combined anterior cruciate and medial collateral ligament injury–a biomechanical study in a goat model. J Orthop Res. 2003;21(6):1124–30.
48. Kanamori A, Sakane M, Zeminski J, Rudy TW, Woo SL. In-situ force in the medial and lateral structures of intact and ACL-deficient knees. J Orthop Sci. 2000,5(6):567–71.
49. Sakane M, Livesay GA, Fox RJ, Rudy TW, Runco TJ, Woo SL. Relative contribution of the ACL, MCL, and bony contact to the anterior stability of the knee. Knee Surg Sports Traumatol Arthrosc. 1999;7(2):93–7.
50. Yoshiya S, Kuroda R, Mizuno K, Yamamoto T, Kurosaka M. Medial collateral ligament reconstruction using autogenous hamstring tendons: technique and results in initial cases. Am J Sports Med. 2005;33(9):1380–5.
51. Zaffagnini S, Bonanzinga T, Marcheggiani Muccioli GM, Giordano G, Bruni D, Bignozzi S, Lopomo N, Marcacci M. Does chronic medial collateral ligament laxity influence the outcome of anterior cruciate ligament reconstruction?: a prospective evaluation with a minimum three-year follow-up. J Bone Joint Surg Br. 2011;93(8):1060–4.
52. Fetto JF, Marshall JL. Medial collateral ligament injuries of the knee: a rationale for treatment. Clin Orthop Relat Res. 1978;132:206–18.
53. Ibrahim SA. Primary repair of the cruciate and collateral ligaments after traumatic dislocation of the knee. J Bone Joint Surg Br. 1999;81(6):987–90.
54. Owens BD, Neault M, Benson E, Busconi BD. Primary repair of knee dislocations: results in 25 patients (28 knees) at a mean follow-up of four years. J Orthop Trauma. 2007;21(2):92–6. https://doi.org/10.1097/BOT.0b013e3180321318.
55. Yeh WL, Tu YK, Su JY, Hsu RW. Knee dislocation: treatment of high-velocity knee dislocation. J Trauma. 1999;46(4):693–701.
56. Halinen J, Lindahl J, Hirvensalo E. Range of motion and quadriceps muscle power after early surgical treatment of acute combined anterior cruciate and grade-III medial collateral ligament injuries. A prospective randomized study. J Bone Joint Surg Am. 2009;91(6):1305–12.
57. Li T, Xiong Y, Zhang Z, Tang X, Chen G, Li Q, Fu WL, Li J. Results of multiple ligament reconstruction after knee dislocation——a prospective study with 95 patients and minimum 2-year follow up. BMC Musculoskelet Disord. 2021;22(1):904. https://doi.org/10.1186/s12891-021-04596-9.
58. Korber SS, Fathi A, Bolia IK, Panish BJ, Benvegnu N, Juhan TW, Weber AE, Argintar EH, Hatch GF. Outcomes of multiligament knee injury treated with versus without internal brace suture augmentation. Eur J Orthop Surg Traumatol. 2024;34(1):303–9. https://doi.org/10.1007/s00590-023-03575-1.
59. Ma W, Yang Y, Ha X. Two-stage ligament reconstruction with remnant preservation as treatment of knee dislocation. BMC Surg. 2023;23(1):371. https://doi.org/10.1186/s12893-023-02271-5.
60. Gensior TJ, Mester B, Achtnich A, Winkler PW, Henkelmann R, Hepp P, Glaab R, Krause M, Frosch K-H, Zellner J, Schoepp C. Anatomic repair and ligament bracing as an alternative treatment option for acute combined PCL injuries involving the posteromedial or posterolateral

corner—results of a multicentre study. Arch Orthop Trauma Surg. 2023;143(12):7123–32. https://doi.org/10.1007/s00402-023-05015-5.

61. Ateschrang A, Döbele S, Freude T, Stöckle U, Schröter S, Kraus TM. Acute MCL and ACL injuries: first results of minimal-invasive MCL ligament bracing with combined ACL single-bundle reconstruction. Arch Orthop Trauma Surg. 2016;136(9):1265–72. https://doi.org/10.1007/s00402-016-2497-6.

MIX
Papier aus verantwortungsvollen Quellen
Paper from responsible sources
FSC® C105338

If you have any concerns about our products, you can contact us on
ProductSafety@springernature.com

In case Publisher is established outside the EU, the EU authorized representative is:
Springer Nature Customer Service Center GmbH
Europaplatz 3, 69115 Heidelberg, Germany

Printed by Libri Plureos GmbH
in Hamburg, Germany